Mrs. M. L. Florence
508 Wilson Av.
Bellingham, Wash

Feminine Forever

Feminine Forever

by *ROBERT A. WILSON*
M.D., F.I.C.S., F.A.C.S., F.A.C.O.G.

Consultant in Obstetrics and Gynecology, Methodist Hospital, Brooklyn, N.Y.; St. Mary's Hospital, Brooklyn, N.Y.; Putnam Community Hospital, Carmel, N.Y.

Published by
M. EVANS AND COMPANY, INC.,
New York,
and distributed in association with
J. B. LIPPINCOTT COMPANY,
Philadelphia *and* New York

To my wife Thelma, *who was predestined to be the cause of one of the greatest biological revolutions in the history of civilization. Her interest in medical research, her capacity to translate theory into reality with its inescapable toil and drudgery, her indomitable courage in times of discouragement, all served to bring to womankind a priceless gift—the elimination of the menopause, woman's physical, mental, and final emancipation.*

Acknowledgments

THE STUDIES UPON which this book is based could never have been brought to culmination without the interest, encouragement and scientific guidance of a physician whose name must remain unknown.

Dr. Edmund R. Marino, Attending Pathologist and Director of Laboratory, Carson C. Peck Memorial Hospital, Brooklyn, New York, has collaborated with me over the years in the development, refinement and extensive clinical testing of the Femininity Index described in this book.

I gratefully acknowledge the help and valuable advice of Mr. Hans Fantel in the preparation of the manuscript.

Mr. Robert A. Wilson, Jr. produced the illustrations, furnished invaluable suggestions and provided much of the dynamism needed in times of discouragement.

Contents

Foreword

No spring nor summer beauty hath such grace
As I have seen in one autumnal face.

With these words John Donne, an ardent admirer of feminine pulchritude, paid a rare tribute to woman's autumnal years rather than to her springtime of puberty or her summer of fertility.

The life history and destiny of each woman are dependent to a great degree on the intensity and duration of her ovarian function. Her femininity encompasses three phases: puberty, the reproductive years, and the climacteric or the menopause. The onset of menstruation outwardly manifests that pubescence is about to end and the reproductive years are at hand. The menopause, the cessation of the menses, heralds the beginning of a change in the way of life from fertility to the end of reproductive potential. The menopause signifies that a woman has climbed a higher rung in her progression through life: the climacteric. Ovarian function subsides, estrogen production declines, and menstrual flow ceases; she is now freed from the responsibilities, the stress, the hazards, and the trials and tribulations of childbirth—but at a price. For most, the effects of estrogen deprivation are physically and emotionally devastating; for a fortunate few the damage is minimal, the scars only slightly visible.

When we consider a woman's biological constitution, and the vicissitudes of her environment, it is clear why she enters the climacteric with uneasy and uncertain tread. She dreads the threat of declining femininity, of waning romance. For her, it may well become a period of emotional irritability and instability. Little wonder, then, that the psychosexual upheaval connected wth this time of life is apt to trigger a train of varied symptoms—one physician stamping these as psychoneurotic, another considering them as menopausal.

Heretofore, the menopause has been regarded as a physiological state, admittedly damaging to the body economy; an inevitable though unwelcome expectation. Doctor Wilson, with messianic zeal, has campaigned for its abolition. His voice is being heard and re-echoed. Like a gallant knight he has come to rescue his fair lady not at the time of her bloom and flowering but in her despairing years; at a time of life when the preservation and prolongation of her femaleness are so paramount. Actually, he is carrying on and extending an approach already established by several pioneering physicians. The long-time management of the menopause, so long neglected by most, was advocated in the past by a few. The way was prepared. Now, Doctor Wilson, with boldness and clarity of purpose, sounds the clarion call, awakening a slumbering profession to a woman's needs and defies the traditional *laissez-faire* of physicians toward the hormonal treatment of the postmenopausal woman.

Feminine Forever is not to be confused with the sexuality and sensuality of Kathleen Winsor's *Forever Amber*. The essence of his book is more in tune with the ideas so succinctly expressed by Simone de Beauvoir when in *The Second Sex* she wrote about the pathetic urgency of those who have staked everything on their femininity to turn back the flight of time. Doctor Wilson shares the optimism of Browning's Rabbi Ben Ezra, "The last of life, for which the first was made."

By throwing down his gauntlet, he challenges the reluctant physician to follow him in providing the hormones that may allow for a smoother transition to the menopausal years ahead. Woman will be emancipated only when the shackles of hormonal deprivation are loosed. Then, she will be capable of obtaining fulfillment without interrupting her quest for a continuum of physical and mental health. Aging need not be equated with calendar years any more than service need be hampered by time. She can grow old with grace and human worth, glowing with the radiance of the turning leaves of fall. Such was Shakespeare's vision when he penned the lines

> *To me, fair friend, you never can be old,*
> *For as you were when first your eye I ey'd*
> *Such seems your beauty still.*

Doctor Wilson, too, recaptures the poetic prophesies of a distant day when he endows woman with her right to be forever feminine.

ROBERT B. GREENBLATT, M.D.
Professor and Chairman
Department of Endocrinology
Medical College of Georgia

Augusta, Georgia
September 27, 1965

A Biological Revolution

AMONG THE NEARLY hundred million women living in the United States today, a select minority, numbering between six and twelve thousand at present are spearheading a new kind of sexual revolution. They are pointing the way to a new biological destiny for every human female.

This book is an invitation to all women to share this adventure.

The women in this pioneer group are different in one vital aspect from any other woman since the beginning of the human race: They will never suffer menopause.

Instead of being condemned to witness the death of their own womanhood during what should be their best years, they will remain fully feminine—physically and emotionally—for as long as they live.

You may have passed them on the street or seen them on the bus. You may have met them at a party, in church, or at the club. Perhaps one of them is working at your office. You can't tell unless you know their age.

But when you find a woman of 50 looking like 30, or a woman of 60 looking—and acting—like 40, chances are that she is one of the lucky ones who have benefited from the new techniques of menopause prevention.

The outward signs of this age-defying youthfulness are a straight-backed posture, supple breast contours, taut, smooth skin on face and neck, firm muscle tone, and that particular vigor and grace typical of a healthy female. At fifty, such women still look attractive in tennis shorts or sleeveless dresses.

To the emotionally mature woman, this physical attractiveness is rarely an end in itself. Rather, it is a subtle psychological means by which she relates to the world around her. While this quality may not be directly erotic, its charm usually derives from a woman's sexual self-confidence. And now, thanks to recent medical advances, it is possible for any woman to retain her sexual appeal along with her sexual vitality throughout later life. By retaining these functions she also safeguards the less direct and more elusive aspects of her total femininity.

The biological revolution that is just now beginning to reach a significant number of women stems from a series of medical discoveries about the chemical causes of menopause—the stoppage of female sexual functions in middle life. Before these discoveries, menopause had been regarded as a normal condition for women at a certain age. As a result, nobody even considered it necessary to understand its causes. Physicians wrongly assumed that age itself was the cause.

When I began my investigations some forty years ago, I realized that very little prior research had been done in this field. Predominantly male, the medical profession had apparently failed to appreciate the menopause as a serious physical and mental syndrome. As a result of this "male provincialism" in medicine, little effort had been made to apply modern research techniques to menopausal problems. It had been the custom to regard menopause as a "natural" occurrence —an inevitable part of woman's fate, and this traditional view still prevails in some medical quarters. Even today, the many dangerous and agonizing symptoms that often accompany a woman's "change of life" are still shrugged off by many otherwise-reputable physicians as nothing but "a state of mind".

This medical attitude, I believe, is dictated by a fairly common type of male indifference to anything exclusively female, except as it affects men. In a male-oriented culture which for centuries has accorded an inferior status to women and condoned their sexual exploitation, a certain lack of empathy with female problems may be expected. Yet it strikes me as particularly unfortunate that something of this anti-feminine attitude still survives in some circles of the medical profession. Added to the aura of irrationality that still surrounds the subject of female sexuality both inside and outside the medical profession, this lack of basic sympathy for women has for many years forestalled serious medical research on menopausal problems.

I realized early in my career as a gynecologist that I could not accept this attitude. The often-severe suffering of my menopausal patients made me regard menopause as a serious medical condition endangering the health and happiness of any woman, and it was in this light that I conducted my research.

In the course of my work, spanning four decades and involving hundreds of carefully documented clinical cases, it became evident that menopause—far from being an act of fate or a state of mind—is in fact a deficiency disease. By way of rough analogy, you might think of menopause as a condition similar to diabetes. Both are caused by lack of a certain substance in the body chemistry. To cure diabetes, we supply the lacking substance in the form of insulin. A similar logic can be applied to menopause—the missing hormones can be replaced.

Although this new concept of menopause has been distressingly slow to find acceptance in the highly tradition-minded medical profession, the following clinical facts are now firmly established.

Menopause is curable. Under proper treatment, nearly all symptoms cease in the vast majority of cases. The bodily changes typical of middle age can be reversed, and sexual functions can be restored, along with a fully feminine appearance. The only sexual function that cannot be restored is fertility.

Menopause is completely preventable. No woman need suffer menopause or any of its symptoms if she receives preventive treatment *before* the onset of menopause.

The bulk of this book is an account of the results attained by therapy of this type. As originator of this form of treatment and one of the earliest practitioners in this field, I am profoundly grateful that good fortune has permitted me to find the key by which any woman can now gain a new dimension of control over her destiny.

I can assert the following as a simple statement of clinical fact: Every woman alive today has the option of remaining feminine forever. No longer need she fret about the cruel irony of women aging faster than men. It is simply no longer true that the sexuality of a woman past forty necessarily declines more rapidly than that of her husband. This alone, I believe, may indefinitely prolong the happiness of millions of families whose marital foundations might otherwise have eroded under the usual psycho-sexual stress of middle life. Quite aside from the purely medical aspects of this therapy, I feel that its ultimate merit lies in the possibility of bringing enrichment and harmony to a woman's marriage at a time in her life when these qualities are especially needful to her.

The medical discoveries cited in this book were, of course, first published in the proper professional journals, including the *Journal of the American Medical*

Association (see Medical Appendix). The therapeutic routines outlined in Chapter 6 have been tested in hundreds of cases, not merely in my own practice but also at Methodist Hospital in Brooklyn, New York, where I have served on the staff for forty-three years.

But, within the topical confines of medical reports, it is rarely possible to treat the broader implications of a subject. In matters of sex, in particular, many doctors prefer to restrict their attention to immediate symptoms. The writing of medical papers in gynecology is often similarly limited. I cannot regard my work as being within such narrow limits.

In my daily contact with patients, I constantly observed the wider ramifications of sex. I could not fail to notice how a woman's awareness of her own femininity completely suffuses her character and how the tragedy of menopause often destroys her character along with her health. Time and again I have pondered how sexuality, in its more indirect manifestations, often determines a woman's sense of her own worth and thus sets the total pattern of her human relations.

I therefore believe that menopause prevention far transcends the purely clinical aspects of the subject. It even transcends any narrow view of sex as such. What is really at stake is a subtle and almost metaphysical factor—a woman's total femininity.

To place the clinical aspect of my discoveries in relation to these broader implications, I decided to present this account of my life's work not in rigidly medical terms but to write this book for those to whom every physician is ultimately responsible—the lay public.

The concept of menopause prevention—after having so long been stymied by indifference and outmoded attitudes—is at last spreading from a relatively small group of enlightened physicians to wider circles of the medical profession.

Clinical reports from many parts of the country and from Europe bear out my own findings with remarkable consistency. Though menopausal treatment by private physicians rarely shows up in medical statistics, it is a safe estimate that the number of sexually restored post-menopausal women in America will pass fourteen thousand in 1967.

Admittedly, this is but a puny fraction of the many millions who might potentially benefit. But these women constitute a significant beginning of a wholly new concept of woman's life.

Our attitudes toward age are changing rapidly as modern medicine increases the average life expectancy. Not too long ago—certainly within my own memory—a woman of forty was regarded as being beyond the most significant years of her life. Certainly, this psychological barrier has been removed. Today a woman in her forties is considered to be in her most active prime. Many women in this age bracket are nowadays at the height of their business and professional careers, and on the domestic scene the image of the young, attractive grandmother is rapidly supplanting the more traditional stereotype of grandmotherhood.

Thirty years ago, when England's monarch abandoned his throne for the love of a woman approaching forty, Mrs. Simpson's age seemed as much of a shock to the world as the royal abdication itself. Were this event to happen today, our attitudes toward her age would be as different as are our attitudes toward royalty.

While the mental barriers to personal fulfillment during the middle years have been removed, the physical barrier of menopause has until now remained immovable for the majority of women. Even for otherwise progressive, emancipated women, the threat of menopause still is a cause of serious anxiety. Yet such fears are now groundless. At last, the physical obstacles to full femininity after forty have given way along with the mental impediments.

In effect, the new medical possibilities double a woman's emotional life span. Forty no longer looms as a dividing line. No longer is her life in danger of being broken in half by "the change". Now at last, her life can be a harmonious continuity not threatened by the sudden disruption of her womanhood but marked by the growth and enrichment of that womanhood.

Psychologically, this knowledge even transforms her younger years. It removes from her thirties the burden of an unspoken fear. She no longer feels the dreadful compulsion to make the years count. She no longer is haunted by the pursuing sense of time running out for her. Thanks to the medical advances detailed in this book, today's woman is the first of her species with *enough* time to fulfill her human potential, both physically and emotionally.

The years added to her womanhood promise in some ways to be her happiest and most meaningful. For during her later years she enjoys a wisdom of experience that young women have yet to acquire. Against this richer background, the possibilities of physical femininity are all the greater and the more enjoyable.

Looking back over my long service as a physician, I take profound satisfaction in knowing that I have helped preserve the health and happiness of thousands of my patients by enabling them to continue their existence *as women* beyond their middle years. With this book, addressed to numberless women whom I shall never see, I hope to spread the awareness of a medical routine that can transform lives.

1

A Woman's Right to Be Feminine

A GIRL BORN in the heyday of the Roman Empire had a life expectancy of about twenty-three years. To be sure, life expectancy is but a statistical abstraction. Obviously many Roman women lived longer. But beyond the age of forty their ranks thinned. With relatively few women living past that point, menopause just wasn't much of a problem in ancient Rome.

In this respect, matters didn't change much for centuries. A visit to any old New England graveyard usually shows a man's grave surrounded by two or three smaller monuments—one for each wife. In pioneer America it was pretty much taken for granted that women wore out young. A man expected to outlive at least one wife and then have to look for another. Menopause rarely troubled these short-lived women. Individual women who outlived the average and suffered serious menopausal effects were simply classified as "ailing females" and could expect little sympathy and no medical help at all.

Even in Victorian times, "Mrs. Average launched her family and then died like a spent skyrocket in her mid-forties," observes Dr. Robert Rutherford, editor of the *Western Journal of Surgery, Obstetrics and Gynecology*. With relatively few long-lived women in the total population, menopause simply wasn't recognized as a serious social problem during most of human history.

Yet a girl born today can expect to live about seventy-five years. The world is filling up with women with a large part of life still ahead of them after menopause.

After lengthening the human lifespan—and particularly the lifespan of women by lessening the risks of pregnancy and childbirth—medical science now faces a new responsibility: it must help women retain their full physical and mental facilities during the extra years added to the average lifespan. In short, menopause must at last be recognized as a major medical problem in modern society. Women, after all, have the right to remain women. They should not have to live as sexual neuters for half their lives. The treatment and cure of menopause thus becomes a social and moral obligation. At this point in history, medical science can no longer evade the responsibility of helping women remain feminine for life.

Along with longevity, the twentieth century has produced a cultural climate that puts a premium on femininity. For better or worse, we live in a world in which sensual vividness has become a pervasive factor. Our media of entertainment—literature, theater, the movies, and television—have completely abandoned traditional restraints. Whether sexual situations are presented with deplorable crudeness or artistic finesse, the fact remains that the entire cultural climate in which we live has become suffused with a heightened sexual awareness. In purely pictorial terms, we are surrounded by alluring women, smiling at us from countless advertising pages or cooing seductively from millions of loudspeakers. Even a simple weather forecast nowadays calls for some ravishing girl on the TV screen to raise the temperature and explain the highs and lows.

In the final line of *Faust*, Goethe speaks of the mystic attraction of the Eternally-Female (*"Das Ewig-Weibliche zieht uns hinan"*). The advertising moguls of the world have freely translated such metaphysics into a simple slogan: "Sex sells." In consequence, women particularly in post-Puritan cultures have had a new role thrust upon them: femininity has become the universal gimmick, the spirit that fires the economy into an ever-growing gross national product.

In its crassest forms, the commercialization of sex is as insulting to true femininity as the Puritan attitude, which regarded feminine attractiveness as downright diabolic. And, like the Puritan attitude, it imposes certain risks and penalties upon women. Where a naturally feminine and profoundly alluring woman in prior times ran the risk of being burned as a witch, modern woman faces the opposite dilemma. To function effectively in a sex-dominated culture, she herself has to be reasonably sexy—that is, confident of her feminine appearance and charm.

This need for distinctive femininity as an indispensable social asset is by no means confined to young girls on a husband hunt. A matron's prestige and a businesswoman's success depend too, at least indirectly, on the body chemistry that enables a woman to attain full femininity, both physically and psychologically. And with the extra years of a longer lifespan, the modern woman understandably longs for ways to retain her invaluable aura of femininity long past the traditional barrier of menopause.

I believe that the emotional liberation of women ranks as one of the greatest contributions to human progress that this century has produced. It is an achievement of the human spirit of perhaps greater long-range significance than space exploration, or any of the other purely technical advances of our time. Yet I am often disturbed at the crassness and blatancy with which women themselves proclaim their sexual liberation. Feminine fashion, for instance, appears to have abandoned the ancient wisdom that concealment is the secret of allure. Speaking from the male point of view, I can only express doubt that the modern woman, frantically emphasizing her physique with tight-fitting stretch pants, really makes herself attractive to any man. The crudely suggestive nomenclature of perfumes—with such labels as "Innuendo," "My Sin," and "Tabu"—certainly makes me sympathize with the girl shown in a recent cartoon in the *Saturday Review*. She plaintively asks at the drugstore: "Don't you have something that just smells nice?"

It may seem trivial to make these points. However, I believe that such matters as dress, grooming, manners, and style of language are as much related to a woman's femininity as her physical attributes. Medically speaking I cannot separate these peripheral factors from a patient's total functioning as a woman. If we are to prolong a woman's femininity by means of medical techniques, I believe that her femininity should be preserved not merely in body but also in spirit. Only then can she function fully as a woman within her particular human context.

If a woman is to understand and fulfill her role in this century, it may help her to be aware of the historical precedents that have led to her present situation. I have observed that the present emphasis on sex in literature, theater, and movies, has led to a devaluation of sex. By falling in with the cheap exhibitionism of commercialized sex—by displaying a glib pseudo-sophistication in dress, manner, and language—many women have themselves contributed to the downgrading of femininity.

I can only hope that this is a passing phase of overreacting to the prohibitions of the past. After all, the change in our attitude toward sex—and women in particular—has come with astonishing speed.

It was less than a century ago that the Rev. Harvey Newcomb epitomized the American attitude toward sex in a sermon to young men: "When you feel any inclination to go abroad in search of forbidden pleasures, I advise you to stay home with your sisters and sing 'Home Sweet Home.'" Another writer of the times suggested that, in households with a grand piano, the legs of the instrument should be covered with skirts for reasons of modesty. I often wondered why he regarded pianos as female.

Such prissy notions were harmful both to men and women, tending to arrest the emotional development of both sexes at the level of adolescence. Yet it was the woman who had to bear the brunt of the grotesque sexphobia that afflicted both England and America during the past three hundred years. Even the most straight-laced Puritan, warily sidestepping the snares of the Evil One, always granted that the sexual impulse *in men* had to be tolerated. Of course, he tried to make sex as unpleasant as possible, to insure himself against the mortal dangers of sinful joy. But the Puritan moralist would grudgingly allow the sexual arousal of men as necessary for the production of children. With women it was different. They didn't need to be aroused for purposes of conception. Consequently, traditional morality looked upon the sexually responsive woman as a wanton creature straight from the maw of hell.

Not until the present century has it been generally accepted that sex fulfills a vital role in human life quite apart from the production of children. Perhaps the most far-reaching change in human society in the twentieth century is this re-classification of sex. Sex no longer has as its aspects the limited alternatives of procreation or sinfulness. It has been recognized as a vastly enriching element that is the key to wholly new dimensions in the development of human personality. This shift of values may prove an important turning point in the culture of the Western world.

Yet the Puritan shadow still hangs over many women, making them either sexually inhibited, or—by way of overcompensation—sexually wanton. Only the woman who sees her femininity in historical context may be able to steer clear of both the restrictiveness of the past and the gross tastelessness of present-day sex emphasis. She will take a realistic measure of her own sexual needs and rights, and this mature self-knowledge will help her cherish and fulfill the best potentials of her feminine role in life.

The elimination of menopause is perhaps the most important technical advance by which women may equip themselves for an enduringly feminine role in modern life. As a physician, it is therefore disconcerting to me that large segments of the medical profession still fail to understand the modern woman's need to remain fully feminine throughout her lengthened lifespan. Certainly, frankness in matters of sex—so characteristic of many areas of modern life—has not yet penetrated into the one realm where the most legitimate need exists for such frankness—the consulting room of the gynecologist. Particularly when the patient's complaint involves menopause in its many symptoms, too many doctors simply dismiss the subject.

One of my patients, a sprightly woman of forty-five suffering the first signs of menopause, had come to me because a friend had told her of my work in menopause therapy.

"Have you discussed your symptoms with your family doctor?" I asked her.

"He couldn't care less!" she shot back with an edge of bitterness in her voice.

This woman's experience reflects the traditional attitude of many physicians, who simply refuse to recognize menopause for what it is—a serious, painful, and often crippling disease. These doctors constantly point to the fact that some women never develop serious menopausal difficulties. From this they conclude that any woman who does suffer severely is merely a hypochondriac. So they refuse to take menopausal complaints seriously.

Because these doctors do not consider menopause as a matter worthy of serious medical concern, it is not likely that they will bother to look up recent findings on the subject. If they did, they would discover that women who "age gracefully" and never develop serious menopausal difficulties are not the rule but the exception. Recent clinical studies show that only fifteen percent of women are so fortunate as to avoid serious suffering during menopause and to retain most of their vitality in the years after. They owe their luck not to general good health but to an unusual hormonal condition.

To regard this exceptional fifteen percent as a

"model" and senselessly penalize the remaining eighty-five percent by refusing to take their plight seriously is nothing short of mindless cruelty. To deny proper medical attention to eighty-five percent of all menopausal women merely because fifteen percent are not in need of such help certainly defies the laws of logic as well as the dictates of human compassion.

Yet one cannot accuse the average practitioner of willful neglect if he fails to treat menopause properly. If he is not yet aware that menopause is a curable disease, caused by a deficiency of estrogen hormones, the doctor could be easily misled by its symptoms.

A patient of mine had been to several doctors before she finally was referred to me. Each of these doctors had treated her most conscientiously and to the best of his knowledge and ability. Because she was suffering from digestive upsets, her family physician referred her to a gastro-intestinal specialist. Despite an extensive series of gastro-intestinal tests, he could find no apparent cause for her symptoms. Naturally, the gastro-intestinal specialist reached the conclusion that the woman was a hypochondriac and that her ailments were largely imaginary. To pacify her, he prescribed a harmless diet, which of course did not help her at all.

This woman was lucky that the gastro-intestinal specialist did not take her seriously. Otherwise he might have recommended exploratory surgery to seek the possible causes of her chronic digestive complaints. This would have been entirely consistent with good practice in the gastro-intestinal field. Nothing in the specialist's training would have alerted him to the fact that the woman's digestive troubles were not gastro-intestinal in origin but a "side effect" of her menopausal condition. When I finally took over the case and prescribed the standard menopausal estrogen therapy, the digestive difficulties ceased as soon as the hormone was restored to pre-menopausal level.

Modern specialization in medicine focuses the doctor's attention on symptoms rather than underlying causes. A woman with serious menopausal complications might shuttle between a dozen different specialists, all treating her different menopausal symptoms with a variety of futile measures. One specialist might be concerned with her headaches and fatigue, another with her disturbed vision, another with her skin condition and drying membranes, and still another with her aching bones and joints, and a psychiatrist might be called in to help the poor woman with her understandable mental depression. Quite likely, not one of these doctors would be aware of menopause as the root of all these manifold difficulties. All the doctors, consequently, would proceed with ineffective treatments of the many symptoms rather than prescribe effective treatment of the single cause. Getting plenty of bills, but no relief, from all her specialist doctors, the distraught woman might soon find herself in a hopeless mental, physical, and financial state.

It is not difficult to explain why so many doctors have a "blind spot" for menopause in their diagnostic vision. One reason, as I have pointed out, is the tradition of regarding menopause as a natural phase of aging rather than a disease. Another reason is that menopausal symptoms are so common that the doctor fails to notice them—even in members of his own family.

One of the patients who had received hormone therapy at Brooklyn's Methodist Hospital moved to another part of the country and sought to continue her estrogen treatment with a local physician. That tradition-minded doctor could not be persuaded that menopause called for anything more than "mental" adjustment. Finally, as the doctor ushered her out of the consulting room she said to him: "All right, doctor, if I can't convince you, go take a look at your own wife."

The catty remark suggests an important truth. If doctors would look upon their middle-aged wives with a keen diagnostic eye, asking themselves more than simply what has happened to the girls they married, they might give more thought to the problems of menopause. Of course, in a doctor's day-to-day contact with his wife, the changes wrought by menopause may not seem very dramatic. But if the doctor has sufficient love or empathy for his wife, he might try to imagine how she feels about the waning of womanhood—to say nothing of the fatigue and pain that nearly all women suffer in those years. If more doctors' personal lives were touched by such sympathy, the medical attitude toward menopause would be revolutionized.

In a paper published in the *Journal of the American*

Geriatrics Society (April, 1962), I suggested that the lack of medical sympathy for menopausal women might simply be due to the fact that most doctors, being male, are themselves immune to the disease. To shock my fellow physicians out of their complacent selfishness, I wrote: "Let us reverse the situation. Suppose the man of medicine noticed his own genitals gradually shrinking year by year. Would he be as indifferent to genital atrophy as he now appears to be? We think not."

The medical attitude concerning menopause may be quite different in the Soviet Union, where the majority of physicians are women. Unfortunately, no data on this culturally interesting point can be found in the available literature. It certainly would be a promising subject for a medical study.

But the most important factor accounting for the diagnostic "blind spot" concerning menopause lies in the limitations of medical training. In his four years in medical school, a student has to assimilate a vast mass of information. Perhaps no more than a single thirty-minute lecture is devoted to menopause during a doctor's entire medical education. This neglect of the subject appears quite justified in the traditional view of menopause as a normal part of aging. "Why bother about something that can't be helped?" is the prevailing logic.

Thanks to the new discoveries, menopause now *can* be helped. It's time the medical profession woke up to this fact. One may hope that the new insights into the nature of menopause will earn the subject a greater share of the medical curriculum. With the health and happiness of half the total population at stake, menopause should certainly rate a prominent place in any doctor's education. Once this educational task is accomplished, women will no longer run the risk of being sent from one specialist to another for ineffective symptomatic treatment while the cause of their condition remains unrecognized. After medical school, the pattern of neglect continues during internship. The young doctor rarely is motivated to think about menopause at all. During my own years as an intern, I never heard menopause mentioned—a fact which I noticed because of an early interest in the subject. But my young colleagues, deeply engrossed in the high drama of witnessing advanced surgery, or tending the emergency room, were hardly aware of this omission. Interns with acute medical minds find themselves pondering such challenging cases as acute leukemia, diabetic coma, malignant hypertension, nephrosis, or chemotherapy for disseminated cancer. In such a mental climate, menopause seems like drab fare indeed.

Later these men enter practice knowing nothing and caring less about the menopausal cases they will doubtless encounter. I know of one physician of this type who, on twenty-two occasions, sent away severely suffering menopausal women with nothing more helpful than his smile and bland assurances.

Against this discouraging background, it seems all

the more fortunate that a fast-growing number of influential physicians are now re-thinking the entire medical approach in the light of recent discoveries and the new possibility of complete cure. Among the pioneers in this field, principal tribute is due to the late Dr. Kost Shelton of Los Angeles. His article, "The use of Estrogen After the Menopause", published in the *Journal of the American Geriatrics Society* (October, 1954), was one of the first beacons of enlightenment in the engulfing sea of ignorance. It should be required reading for every doctor seriously interested in the health, happiness, femininity, and dignity of his women patients.

I have consistently stressed the importance of medical attitude as much as medical technique in respect to the menopause problem. After all, the relationship between a woman and her physician is a deeply personal one, and what is involved in menopausal treatment is not merely the administration of hormones but the preservation of a total personality.

I believe that every emotionally mature, cultivated man recognizes at some time in his life that the most engaging and most deeply meaningful of all human qualities are expressed in the physical and spiritual grace of a truly feminine woman. This is the reason why men fall in love.

A man always marries Helen of Troy or Aphrodite—an angelic, ethereal creature whose beauty was sung by poets of the past. And through the daily round of shopping for groceries, drying dishes, or tending babies, he stubbornly clings to the image of his wife as a mysterious, dreamlike incarnation of some superb fancy. Men are incredibly loyal in this way, providing they get a little cooperation from their wives in supporting this gallant fantasy.

Human love at any civilized level has less to do with mating as such than with the fundamental recognition of the surpassing fineness of what is truly feminine.

Women, of course, fall in love too—but for somewhat different reasons. What they seek in men will be discussed in a later chapter. But for a man, a truly feminine woman is the idol that inspires his own capacity to lift himself beyond his ordinary limits. Desire, to be sure, is part of this drive. But the femininity of a woman also evokes in man the capacity for adoration.

This, of course, is the root of the great tradition of chivalry and romantic love in our civilization. Whatever contemporary sneers may be aimed at the romantic concept of love, the fact persists that romance is still the mainspring of motivation—even to the outwardly blasé sophisticates of the twentieth century. It remains the common man's only path beyond his commonness, and the uncommon man's impetus toward whatever heights he may reach. Even the most prosaic among us experience the awareness of an ennobling presence from a truly feminine and gracious woman. The man who may cherish such a woman as his own is fortunate indeed. For him, the world is not well lost for love, but well gained for it.

It is my profound hope that this book, by pointing to recent discoveries in the field of menopause therapy, may serve to prolong for many women—and for the men who love and admire them—that wonderfully happy aura of love and adoration that full femininity inspires.

2

Must Women Tolerate Castration?

WHENEVER I SPEAK of menopause as castration, some shocked nice-Nellies of either sex—a good many of them doctors—protest that I am overstating the case. But castration, I believe, is the proper term for a syndrome depriving a person of his (or her) sexual functions. It makes no difference whether castration is brought about by removing the genital organs with a knife—as in the surgical removal of the ovaries—or whether the ovaries shrivel up and die as the result of menopause. In either case, the effect is the same: the woman becomes the equivalent of a eunuch.

Castration is a drastic event that affects the entire body. Let the evidence speak for itself:

In all but fifteen percent of menopausal women, the following symptoms develop in varying degrees: the tissues dry out, the muscles weaken, the skin sags. The bones, because of the hormonal deficiency, become brittle and porous, easily fractured. The weakening of the bones often leads to an increasingly hunchbacked condition as the years go by, known as "dowager's

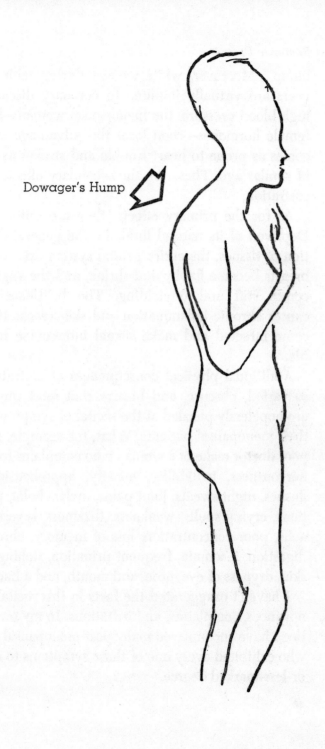

Dowager's Hump

hump." Moreover, while women during their fertile years are virtually immune to coronary disease and high blood pressure, the menopausal woman—lacking female hormones—soon loses this advantage and becomes as prone to heart trouble and strokes as a man of similar age. These are the secondary effects of her castration.

As for the primary effects, they are quite simple. Deprived of its natural fluids by the general desiccation of tissues, the entire genital system dries up. The breasts become flabby and shrink, and the vagina becomes stiff and unyielding. The brittleness often causes chronic inflammation and skin cracks that become infected and make sexual intercourse impossible.

Additional physical consequences of castration are so varied, obscure, and bizarre that most physicians are hopelessly puzzled at the recital of symptoms from their menopausal patients. What, for example, can the poor doctor make of a woman who complains to him of nervousness, irritability, anxiety, apprehension, hot flushes, night sweats, joint pains, melancholia, palpitations, crying spells, weakness, dizziness, severe headache, poor concentration, loss of memory, chronic indigestion, insomnia, frequent urination, itching of the skin, dryness of eye, nose, and mouth, and a backache?

I haven't exaggerated the facts in this recital of annoyances, complaints, and irritations. In my own practice I have encountered many post-menopausal women who exhibited every one of these symptoms to a more-or-less-marked degree.

The effects of menopausal castration, as is evident from this list of symptoms, are by no means confined to the sexual organs. Because the chemical balance of the entire organism is disrupted, menopausal castration amounts to a mutilation of the whole body. I have known cases where the resulting physical and mental anguish was so unbearable that the patient committed suicide.

While not all women are affected by menopause to this extreme degree, no woman can be sure of escaping the horror of this living decay. Every woman faces the threat of extreme suffering and incapacity.

I submit that this is a condition intolerable to modern women. Such waste of human life and happiness cannot be justified either medically or philosophically. Least of all can it be justified by sheer ignorance. Despite the conspiracy of silence surrounding the subject, most women are well aware of the extent to which menopause cripples them. Literally, they feel it in their bones, in their minds, and their hearts. A show of bravery might mask their distress for several years until the symptoms become so obvious that even the most valiant woman can no longer hide the fact that she is, in effect, no longer a woman, but a neuter. Ultimately, not even valor offers escape from this physical reality. What we must learn is that there is no need for either valor or pretense. The need is for hormones.

Most of my private patients consulted me at the first signs of menopausal discomfort, early enough to be cured by intensive hormone therapy. And in recent years, a growing percentage of women came for such treatment even before menopause. For these wise women, no symptoms ever developed. But as a consultant in gynecology to Methodist Hospital in Brooklyn, I have had ample opportunity to witness the terrible results of prolonged menopausal neglect. I have seen untreated women who had shriveled into caricatures of their former selves. Some had lost as much as six inches of height due to pathological bone changes caused by lack of estrogen. Others suffered sweeping metabolic disturbances that literally put them in mortal danger.

Though the physical suffering from menopausal effects can be truly dreadful, what impressed me most tragically is the destruction of personality. Some women, when they realize that they are no longer women, subside into a stupor of indifference. Even so, they are relatively lucky. The most heartbreaking cases, I feel, are those sensitive women who witness their own decline with agonizing self-awareness.

I remember particularly one of my hospital patients, an artistically gifted woman of about fifty-five who showed me some of the charcoal drawings she had done. For lack of a model, she sometimes sketched herself in the mirror. One of these self-portraits— evidently an old one—showed her as a handsome, sturdy woman in her thirties. Then, with an anguished smile, she handed me another sketch.

"That one I did just the other day," she said sadly.

The picture showed a shrunken hag. That's how she saw herself through her own implacable artist's eyes.

The sheer pity of such tragic self-knowledge left me speechless. What that woman must have suffered in comparing the two pictures! And to make the irony the more bitter, the suffering was needless. Early therapy could have halted her decline.

It would be pointlessly horrifying to recount the most tragic cases of menopausal complications I have encountered. They are, after all, extremes. It may be far more useful to focus attention on those women who suffer almost no discernible outward symptoms, but nevertheless suffer serious disruption and disabilities in their post-menopausal years. To illustrate such a situation, I deliberately chose Mrs. G.—not because her case is typical, but because, on the contrary, it is in some ways extraordinary. Here is a woman with everything in her favor: good looks, comparative wealth, an understanding husband, intelligence, education, and—except for menopause itself—basic good health. In short, here is a woman on whom menopause might be expected to have the least effect. Even so, a serious crisis developed.

Mrs. G.'s appearance certainly gave no clue to her difficulties. A handsome, ash-blond woman with a trim figure and an exquisite face, dressed in a stylishly tailored suit, she projected an aura of charm and elegance. Her pleasant, assured manner suggested a gracious hostess or a suave business executive. Yet beneath the carefully maintained façade, Mrs. G. was deeply troubled.

As a young girl, some twenty years earlier, she had

45

been a highly competent executive secretary in a Wall Street brokerage firm. She was successful in yet another way: she married the boss. It was a remarkably happy marriage, and, for two decades, Mrs. G. was busy running her home in suburban Connecticut and bringing up her three children.

"Our house was a sort of neighborhood center," she recalled with a smile. "The children brought over their friends in the afternoon, and my husband brought over his friends in the evening. Frankly, I liked being in the middle of all this activity."

Then her smile vanished.

"The house is empty now," she said in a toneless voice.

When the last of her three boys was packed off to college, Mrs. G. secretly rejoiced. Now at last she would have the freedom to travel and see something of the world. Her husband, of course, would have to stay with his business. The temporary separation didn't frighten either of them. Though deeply fond of each other, Mrs. G. and her husband had not maintained a close physical relationship for several years, and they were able to contemplate each other's absence with equanimity.

She set off for Europe, summering in Switzerland and living in the Balearic Islands during the cold part of the year. Her wealth provided her with every comfort, and her attractive looks insured her against loneliness.

She volunteered no information about her sex life

during her stay abroad. Her innate sense of tact obviously disposed her toward reticence. But I considered this facet as clinically important, and in response to my direct question, she frankly recounted several brief and apparently quite satisfactory love affairs. Her menopausal condition evidently had not then hindered her in that respect.

Throughout this period, Mrs. G. maintained a lively and cordial correspondence with her husband and children, who occasionally visited her in Europe. Outwardly, at least, her life seemed enviable indeed.

Yet, like so many menopausal women, Mrs. G. developed an odd restless melancholy.

"I seemed to be living in a vacuum," she recalled. "My life seemed to be over. I'd sit on a marvelous hotel terrace in Luzern, looking out on the Alps, surrounded by friends. And yet I'd feel despondent."

Mrs. G. decided that the novelty of travel had worn off. She needed a new focus of interest. As she rummaged through her memories, her earlier career at the brokerage firm seemed to her an exciting and happy time. She returned to America resolved to find a job.

"And," she added almost shyly, "I wanted my husband back. I wanted to be a working wife. Maybe I felt that was the way to be young again."

It was during her attempted re-entry into marriage and work that she came face-to-face with the realities faced by thousands of menopausal women. Finding a job was no problem—thanks to her excellent social connections. Her familiarity with stock transactions combined with her personal charm and tact abundantly qualified her to handle customer relations in a brokerage house. But at the office, ranked as a "junior" executive, she found herself in competition with the younger, more vigorous group that set the pace. Much of her energy had been spent upon the bearing and raising of her children. Despite her talents, the job was a strain. Yet she knew that re-establishing herself in her profession was for her the only escape from ennui. Her pride and self-respect depended on her success.

The symptoms of menopause grew more severe under the stress of her new situation. She was constantly tired and beset by severe backaches. Still another element added to her distress: with increasing physical discomfort, she had become sexually insecure.

Like so many women who have ceased to menstruate, she felt a subconscious need to prove her femininity. She wanted to resume normal relations with her husband, but her increasingly nervous disposition and irritability kept him at a distance. In her emotional agitation, she was no longer able to accept his remoteness, however cordial he remained toward her.

Her anxieties mounted—many of them totally irrational. When Mrs. G. first came to me, she felt sure that she was about to lose both her husband and her job. The world held no hope and no meaning for her.

"What am I good for now?" she asked. "I hardly have enough energy to get myself to the office in the morning. So it's no wonder my husband no longer bothers to come home in the evening."

It was frankly painful to me to hear a basically capable and still attractive woman speak dispairingly of her "worthlessness."

A less disciplined, more emotional woman than Mrs. G. might under such conditions suffer a severe nervous breakdown. But Mrs. G., thanks to her high intelligence and basic will to succeed, was easily persuaded to try estrogen therapy.

I was frankly doubtful at the time whether hormones alone would be able to lift Mrs. G. from her depression. Very likely, I thought, a combination of hormone therapy and psychiatric counseling might be needed. But within three weeks, it was evident that the mire of anxieties into which she had sunk was simply a menopausal syndrome, amenable to purely physical treatment.

After less than a month of taking estrogen in fairly high concentration, her fears and pains had vanished. Along with her energy and vitality, she regained so much self-confidence, charm, and cheerfulness that— as she told me some time later—she no longer needed to worry about her marriage. Her restored capacities had created the emotional and physical conditions for a new rapprochement between the two marriage partners.

I have described the case of Mrs. G. at considerable length because it represents a situation faced by so many prosperous, upper-middle-class women in their

middle years. The status of such women in the modern
world makes the dilemma of menopause more distressing than ever. Like Mrs. G., many such women com-
pete with men for personal success in business and
industry, taking on responsibilites that have been
spared to women of earlier times. Their longer lifespan
allows them to pursue two careers in one lifetime: one
as mother, the other in business and the professions.
But to fulfill this strenuous dual role, women like Mrs.
G. depend on full retention of their physical capacities. Their mode of life simply does not allow for the
disruptions caused by menopause.

It is barbaric to expect that today's woman—just
because she lives longer—must tolerate castration during what should be her best years. Yet this is precisely
the attitude maintained by those who still insist
that menopause—and the resultant castration—is a
natural consequence of age.

Unquestionably, menopause is related to age. But
the process of aging must be seen in a new perspective.
After all, since modern medicine has lengthened the
lifespan, modern medicine must also adjust the *rate of
aging* to fit the longer life. The general public and the
medical profession have yet to see the simple logic of
this demand. Without adjustment of the aging rate,
long life is an unnatural burden to a woman. With
such an adjustment, long life can indeed be an inex-
pressibly precious and wonderful gift.

The normal, natural, harmonious aging rate with
respect to lifespan is found in the example of a healthy

man. A man remains male as long as he lives. Age does not rob him of his sexual appetite nor of the means of satisfying it. Throughout life he retains his appreciation of a charming girl or a handsome woman, and along with it, a certain liveliness of outlook and level of motivation in other areas that make him function fully and responsibly as a human being. True, his supply of sex hormones diminishes over the years, but his sexuality decreases gradually. No abrupt crisis has to be faced. A man's life proceeds in smooth continuity. His feeling of self remains unbroken.

How different is the fate of woman. Though modern diets, cosmetics, and fashions make her outwardly look even younger than her husband, her body ultimately betrays her. It destroys her womanhood during her prime. At the very moment when she is most able and eager to enjoy her achievements, her femininity—the very basis of her selfhood—crumbles in ruin. But now, at last, medicine offers a practical escape from this fateful dilemma.

With estrogen therapy, the basic handicap of women with respect to men—their fast and painful aging process—is overcome. Women now need not age faster than men. If a woman's body is furnished through pills with the needed estrogen (no longer supplied by her own ovaries), her rapid physical decline in post-menopausal years is halted. Her body retains its relative youthfulness just as a man's does.

While the main objective of estrogen therapy is to slow down the aging rate and to assure the general systemic health of post-menopausal women, the distinctly sexual benefits of estrogen treatment should not be underrated. It seems perfectly obvious that good general health predisposes a woman—no less than a man—to a more active sex life regardless of chronological age.

Again the topic must be viewed in the larger perspective of the realities of modern life. In earlier times, living a simple life with limited knowledge, a woman may have reached the height of her personal development in her early twenties. Today, by contrast, we live in a civilization so complex and diversified that it takes almost forty years for a woman to attain the deeper self-knowledge that enriches her personal relationship. Her emotional maturity could make her marriage even more meaningful in the middle period of life than it had been during her youth. This is especially true of intelligent, educated women with a wide range of awareness. For those with the greatest capacity of mind and heart take the longest to reach their full personal potential. It seems ironically cruel that such a woman's precious femininity is abridged by menopause at almost precisely the moment when sex could be more rewarding to her than ever before.

It has been argued that the extension of a woman's femininity by means of estrogen is "interfering with nature." One might counter such objections by asking whether curing the measles—or any other disease—is also interfering with nature. If so, the art of medicine as a whole would have to be abandoned.

I have never been able to elicit from these glib critics whether they consider "interfering with nature" merely inadvisable or outright immoral, and, if so, for what reasons. If such arguments were carried through, mankind would have to give up all efforts at healing, along with, for example, all types of farming—another form of interfering with nature. It is noteworthy, by the way, that the very origin of human civilization lies in the kind of interference with nature that led to the development of agriculture. Similarly, I believe that the development of higher possibilities of human life lies in the utilization of our medical knowledge.

From a purely biologic point of view, estrogen therapy can hardly be regarded as altering the natural state of life. On the contrary, as we have pointed out before, it merely *restores* a natural harmony between the rate of aging and life expectancy, a harmony that has been disturbed by the lengthened lifespan of modern women. It is the case of the untreated woman—the prematurely aging castrate—that is unnatural. The common occurrence is not necessarily the normal one. The mere fact that such women castrates are prevalent —and getting more so every day as the world fills up with older women—does not make them biologically natural.

Estrogen therapy doesn't *change* a woman. On the contrary: *it keeps her from changing.* Therapy does not alter the natural hormone balance. Rather, it *restores* the total hormone pattern to the normal, premenopausal level. Whether this is interfering with nature or restoring nature is a moot point. The results speak for themselves.

So much for the medical side of the argument. If the question is to be examined on philosophic grounds, I rest my case on the simple contention that castration is a bad thing and that every woman has the right— indeed, the duty—to counteract the chemical castration that befalls her during her middle years. Estrogen therapy is a proven, effective means of restoring the normal balance of her bodily and psychic functions throughout her prolonged life. It is nothing less than the method by which a woman can remain feminine forever.

3

A Woman's Chemistry

THE BODY IS an unfathomed wonder. In exploring the human organism, medical scientists marvel at its harmony and intricacy of design. In comparison to his own body, man's most advanced machines seem like clumsy toys.

To a large extent, the working of the body is still hidden from human knowledge. How the cells arrange themselves to form the organism, how they "know" their specialized jobs in different organs, how growth takes place and heredity ties the bond between succeeding generations—all this is still a mystery. Neither medicine nor biology, in fact, even has an adequate definition for life.

Yet in the past decades, great progress has been made in deciphering the chemistry of the individual organs and isolating the crucial substances responsible for the functioning of these organs. Through investigations into the chemistry of the female sex organs we have arrived at a new understanding of femininity.

This approach to femininity in terms of hormones

should not be construed as an attempt to reduce womanhood to a chemical formula. A woman's secret lies in her human individuality—a realm far beyond the reach of science. But the new insights into the chemistry of the female organism help provide the conditions under which essential womanhood may reach its full unfolding.

One of the paramount medical events of this century was the discovery of the chemical substances produced by the ovaries. Known collectively as "female sex hormones," these substances are responsible for the physical and, to a large degree, the psychological hallmarks of womanhood. Being essential to the over-all chemical balance of the female organism, these hormones also play a key role in a woman's general state of health.

Until some forty years ago it was generally believed that the ovaries had but one function: to act as a storage bin for eggs and to release one egg every twenty-eight days. But in 1923, Drs. Edgar Allen and Edward A. Doisy—two American researchers—discovered that the ovaries also function as a chemical factory. So far-reaching was this discovery that Dr. Doisy was awarded the Nobel Prize for his work. Later research proved that the ovaries produce two distinct hormones, known as estrogen and progesterone, which pour into the bloodstream and are carried to every part of the body.

Before describing the action of these hormones, it may be helpful to outline briefly the anatomy of the female sex organs. In contrast to the sex organs of a man, the woman's reproductive equipment is almost entirely internal and invisible. The only outer part is the vulva, consisting of two pads of flesh that protect the opening of the vagina. The vagina itself is a muscular canal about five inches long. It receives the man's penis during copulation, vents menstrual waste from the womb, and provides passage for the baby to the outside world. The vagina is lined with a mucous membrane, which—as we shall see later—provides valuable clues to a woman's hormone balance.

At its upper end, the vagina leads into the womb, or uterus—a pear-shaped, muscular organ, about four inches long, that hangs supported by ligaments in the lower abdomen between the large, flaring hip-bones. The lower part of the uterus protruding into the vagina is known as the cervix. The function of the uterus is to provide a safe shelter in which the fertilized egg may develop and the embryo be nourished until birth. The uterus is lined with a layer of tissue called the endometrium, which changes considerably during the different phases of the menstrual cycle.

From each side of the uterus, two snake-like ducts—called the Fallopian tubes—lead toward the ovaries. The upper end of these tubes flares out like the horn of a trumpet and has small finger-like projections to steer the eggs released by the ovaries into the ducts. Inside, the Fallopian tubes are lined with tiny hairlike structures which sweep the eggs down into the uterus.

The most crucial part of the entire female sexual apparatus is the ovaries themselves—two almond-shaped structures about one and one half inches long, an inch wide, and half an inch thick, whitish in color, and surrounded by a glistening membrane called the

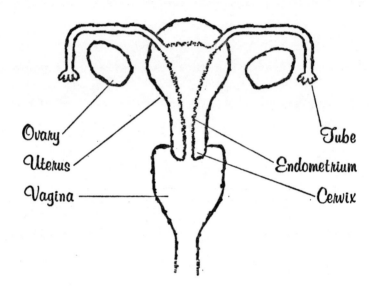

tunica. They are held by ligaments at the left and right sides of the uterus.

Surprisingly, the ovaries of a newborn girl already contain fully formed eggs—about half a million of them. (Of these only about 400 will actually reach maturity and be released during ovulation; the rest will die.) This may seem a rather excessive number of potential babies, but the number appears small in comparison to the potential offspring of the male. Each drop of male seminal fluid contains many millions of sperms. Nature is generous indeed in her assurance of fertility.

Each of the microscopically small eggs in the ovary is packaged in a tiny sac called a follicle. This follicle is lined with layers of special cells called theca and granulosa cells. These are the chemical factories that produce estrogen.

All of these structures work together as a team, co-ordinated by signals transmitted through the female sex hormones. And, although the sexual mechanism was originally designed for purposes of reproduction, the same chemical agents also play a vital part in the non-reproductive—that is, the chiefly psychological—aspects of sex.

The basic rhythm that underlies every woman's life is the menstrual cycle. Each month, a number of follicles enlarge, and one of them ruptures. It then throws its tiny egg into the waiting fingers of the Fallopian tubes. If the woman has had sexual intercourse shortly before that time, the egg may come into head-on collision with one of the millions of male sperms wiggling their way upward in the genital tract. Fusing into each other, egg and sperm preform the *elemental act of creation.* A new being comes into existence, combining the heredities of father and mother. The new embryo then slides downward into the uterus where the richly engorged uterine lining has prepared a cozy place for the developing baby.

If no male sperm happens to be rambling about in the female genitals, the egg remains unfertilized.

When this fact is chemically signaled to the uterus, the womb breaks up the lining it had prepared for the reception of the new baby. The unfertilized egg is eventually swept downward along with the dismantled lining. This is the monthly menstrual discharge. The cycle then begins anew. During her lifetime, as was mentioned before, a woman discharges about 400 of her total stock of half a million eggs.

The chemical key to all these events resides in the female sex hormones secreted by the ovary. When the egg breaks out of its follicle (about midway in the menstrual cycle) it makes quite a tear in the tunica—the covering membrane of the ovary. Some women can actually feel this happen and experience pain at the midpoint of the menstrual cycle. At times this also results in a certain amount of internal bleeding.

A remarkable process follows this monthly rupture of the ovary. The scar tissue of the internal wound turns into a yellow gland—the corpus luteum, producing progesterone. This hormone causes the uterus to preserve the thick lining prepared for the reception of the fertilized egg. If pregnancy results, the corpus luteum keeps making progesterone, the uterine lining remains, and no menstruation takes place. But if the egg remains unfertilized, the corpus luteum dies after a period of about twelve to fourteen days, and the progesterone supply is shut off. The sharp decline of progesterone signals to the uterus that its preparations for a child were in vain. No baby was conceived. The uterus responds to this hormone message by tearing down the interior that was to receive the embryo. The menstrual flow follows—as one medical writer describes it—"the funeral of the unconceived child."

But nature never mourns a lost chance. Instead, it gets busy on the next project. No sooner has the menstrual flow ceased than another hormonal command is received. In response to this command, the follicles in

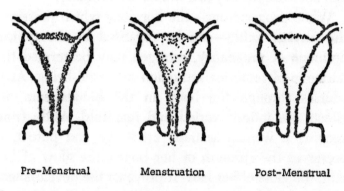

Pre-Menstrual Menstruation Post-Menstrual

the ovaries again secrete increasing amounts of estrogen.

This estrogen consists of a group of substances, such as 17-beta-estradiol, estrone, and several others. But for our purposes we can lump them together under the single name of estrogen. One function of estrogen is to "tell" the uterus to start building up another thick lining for what may be the next baby. But as the estrogen travels through the bloodstream it reaches virtually every part of the body and influences many organs. This is the reason why estrogen is so closely related not merely to the sexual functions but to the general health.

Estrogen as produced by the egg-sacs in the ovaries, for the most part, does not act directly upon the various cells of the body. Before it becomes effective, it must undergo one more process. It passes in the bloodstream through the liver and is chemically changed into compounds called conjugated estrogens (among them estrone and estriol). It is in this form that estrogen becomes the key to a woman's femininity.

While progesterone—the hormone which preserves the uterine lining—can be regarded as the typical hormone of pregnancy, estrogen may be termed the hormone of feminine attraction and well-being. As it courses through the body in the bloodstream, its effects are indeed varied and manifold. Aside from keeping a woman sexually attractive and potent, it preserves the strength of her bones, the glow of her skin, the gloss of her hair. It prevents the development of high blood pressure, heart disease, and strokes. It tends to prevent diabetes and diseases of the urinary bladder, it keeps the kidneys from wasting or losing salt in the urine—a vital matter in the regulation of tissue fluids throughout the body. And this is only a very partial and sketchy list of estrogen functions.

Through an ingenious mechanism by which estrogen acts on the pituitary gland at the base of the brain, it has a direct effect on a woman's emotional state. To a woman, estrogen acts as the carrier of that mysterious life force that motivates work, study, ambition, and that marvelous urge toward excellence that inspires the best of human beings.

Granted, the achievement of any woman cannot be attributed to estrogen alone—estrogen cannot command the fickle element of plain luck. Even with an abundance of estrogen, she still has to cope with the vicissitudes of existence—heredity, accident, environment, childhood training, financial status, and so forth. But at least estrogen puts her in a position where she can take full advantage of whatever lucky breaks come her way. No matter what her particular sphere of activity may be—in the home, in business, in the arts or professions—a woman cannot live up to her opportunities unless she has her full quota of estrogen.

Recent research on chemical influences on the brain indicates that our emotional states—happiness, depression, etc.—depend to a surprisingly large extent on our blood chemistry. To be sure, the outer events of our lives affect our moods. But basic temperament is governed largely by our cerebral metabolism—chemical actions within the brain. Though details of these chemical processes still remain to be explored, clinical observation establishes beyond doubt that certain drugs act as "psychic energizers." Mood-changing drugs are being used increasingly in the treatment of psychological disorders, ranging from mild depression to severe psychosis. My own observation leads me to conclude that—except in cases of some acute emotional shock—women with an ample supply of estrogen in their blood are not likely to develop psychological difficulties calling for the use of such psychic energizers. Estrogen itself acts as a natural energizer to both mind and body. Women rich in estrogen tend to have a certain mental vigor that gives them self-confidence, a sense of mastery over their destiny, the ability to think out problems effectively, resistance to mental and physical fatigue, and emotional self-control. Their emotional reactions are proportional to the occasion. They neither over-react hysterically, nor do they tend toward apathy. They are, as a rule, capable of facing the world with a healthful relaxed attitude and thereby able to enjoy their daily life. They are seldom depressed. Irrational crying spells are virtually unknown among them. In a family situation, estrogen makes women adaptable, even-tempered, and generally easy to live with. Consequently, a woman's estrogen carries significance beyond her own well-being. It also contributes toward the happiness of her family and all those with whom she is in daily contact.

Even frigidity in women, a problem generally supposed to be purely psychological, has been shown to be related to estrogen deficiency. The estrogen-rich woman, as a rule, is capable of far more generous and satisfying sexual responses than women whose femininity suffers from inadequate chemical support.

This fact led to the erroneous conclusion that estrogen increases a woman's sexual desire. Some women have actually refused much-needed estrogen treatment for fear of being turned into nymphomaniacs, unable to turn down any male invitation. Such fears are entirely groundless. No woman's morals were ever threatened by estrogen.

At the root of this mistaken fear of uncontrollable

promiscuity is a basic confusion between sexual responsiveness and sexual desire. It is nothing but a quaint, old-fashioned superstition to suppose that a fully-sexed woman capable of complete sexual response is likely to go astray in search of improper adventures. This is the kind of fiction invented by sex-hating Puritan males. Presumably it had its origin in the fact that such men in previous centuries found their main sexual satisfactions not in the home but in brothels, and they concluded from the businesslike competence of the prostitutes that sexual adeptness goes hand in hand with promiscuity. In fact, there is no connection between the two. On the contrary, an estrogen-rich woman capable of being physically and emotionally fulfilled by her husband or lover is least likely to go afield in search of casual encounters.

Even chemically, there is a distinct opposition between responsiveness and indiscriminate lust. While estrogen aids responsiveness, it takes a chemically *opposite* hormone-androgen to stimulate the libido. Androgen is basically a male hormone, though small amounts of it are normally present in the female and essential to her health. If a woman—due to some pathological condition—has an excess of androgen, her voice deepens and her clitoris (the small projection in her outer genitals) becomes enlarged. Also, her sexual desire increases. For this reason, androgen has been misused as an aphrodisiac. Irresponsible men have secretly fed androgen to young girls to prepare them for a seduction.

This is indeed a criminal act, for the dangers of androgen to a woman are considerable. I have seen cases where excessive doses of androgen had transformed women into hairy creatures with coarse, dark skin and croaking voices. Tragic events of this type have given many people false ideas about hormones. "But doctor, won't it make hair grow all over me?" women asked me when I suggested hormone therapy. The mere mention of the word "hormone" made them think of monstrous malformations. They did not realize that there are many different kinds of hormones with different effects.

The point I wish to stress is that estrogen, unlike some other hormones, has almost no undesirable side effects. It is not an aphrodisiac. No woman, I repeat, is in danger of losing her sexual self-control due to estrogen therapy. Because it invigorates the female sex organs and the total personality, estrogen tends to make sex more enjoyable—regardless of age. But it does not stimulate sexual aggressiveness.

Only in certain special situations may estrogen affect the libido. For example, in an undersexed married woman with small breasts and an undeveloped vagina, the fuller development of these organs resulting from estrogen therapy is sometimes accompanied by an increase in libido. Similarly, in post-menopausal women who have long abstained from sexual intercourse because of physical difficulties caused by menopause, the removal of these physical impediments by estrogen also restores normal sexual appetite. Finally, in slow-developing adolescent girls, estrogen helps to establish normal sexual maturation.

It should be noted that, in these cases, the increase of libido is not *directly* stimulated by estrogen but results from a change in mental attitude toward sex following the restoration of normal body functions.

Still another misconception concerning hormone therapy is the notion that estrogen predisposes toward cancer. The truth is exactly the opposite. There is increasing evidence that estrogen has a preventive effect on breast and genital cancers. In 1962, the *Journal of the American Medical Association* reported on one of my studies, in which a group of 304 women, aged forty to seventy, had been treated with estrogen for periods up to twenty-seven years. Given normal odds, as established by medical statistics, eighteen cases of cancer—either of the breast or the uterus—would normally be expected in this group. Instead, not a single case of cancer occurred!

The most likely explanation of this astonishing result—actual prevention of cancer of the uterine lining—is that estrogen therapy, by restoring menstruation in post-menopausal women maintains one of the most important features of internal hygiene. The monthly flow serves as a kind of internal bath, washing out the womb. Congested tissues—a possible starting point for cancer—continue to be washed away at regular intervals. They don't get a chance to build up along the uterine lining where they might—due to menopausal inactivity and stagnation—undergo malignant change. Statistically, there is evidence that women who stay estrogen-rich throughout their lives will remain happily cancer-poor.

Among all the patients to whom I administered prolonged estrogen therapy I encountered only a single case of uterine cancer, and that particular woman was a referral from another physician and had apparently begun estrogen therapy too late to gain the benefit of its cancer-preventive effect.

The menstrual flow, which most women regard as such a confounded nuisance, thus appears to be an important clause in nature's health insurance policy. As long as a woman menstruates naturally—i.e., before menopause—the flow lessens the likelihood of cancer of the uterine lining to a significant degree. And after the beginning of menopause, she can keep her "cancer insurance" in force by continuing to menstruate as the the result of estrogen therapy.

Now that we have outlined the central importance of estrogen in the chemistry of the female organism, it is easy to see why the loss of estrogen due to menopause is indeed a surpassing tragedy, and why the replacement of estrogen is essential to continued good health and happiness. The specific clinical procedures for counteracting the effects of menopause on the body's estrogen balance are described in Chapter 6. To realize the full significance of those techniques, it is important to understand the relationship between estrogen and over-all hormone balance. This is the topic of the following chapter.

4

A Woman's Body

A WOMAN'S BODY is the key to her fate. This stark assertion does not reflect an unduly carnal point of view. On the contrary; my work as a gynecologist has made me well aware of the extent to which psychic factors shape a woman's personality and determine her health. But to a woman, physique is a more decisive factor than to a man. Since husband, marriage, and children are the fundamental anchor points of her life, her physical, social, and psychological fulfillment all depend on one crucial test: her ability to attract a suitable male and to hold his interest over many years.

Mere physical attractiveness, of course, is no substitute for other feminine qualities, such as a girl's charm or a wife's devotion. Ultimately, in fact, these non-physical qualities contribute more to the content and durability of a marriage than physical endowments. But nearly every woman senses instinctively that, no matter what "other" qualities she may possess, initial physical rapport with her lover, suitor, or husband is necessary to prepare the ground for the unfolding of those other qualities. In short, a woman's physical appeal is her starting capital in the venture of life—the "ante" which lets her into the game.

Physical attractiveness should not be confused with beauty in the purely visual sense. Almost any man will agree that even a homely girl can be delightful if endowed with a certain quality of physical femininity. This quality, indefinable in itself, is a composite of bodily grace, shapeliness, and the emotional and mental correlates that so often result from a healthy body. In short, while femininity is not purely physical, it stems from certain physical prerequisites. As we shall see, these are determined directly by the amount of estrogen in the body.

The growth of a woman's body from childhood to maturity provides clear insight into the crucial role of estrogen in its development.

During childhood, the still-inactive ovaries of a girl do not secrete significant amounts of estrogen. As a result, the girl's sexual organs remain undeveloped. The chest is flat and the uterus looks like a tiny upturned jar, only about one to two inches long. Doctors performing their first abdominal surgery on children are often amazed at the smallness of this organ in prepubertal girls.

The girl-child cannot be considered physically female. With her sexual organs non-functioning and without estrogen—the key to bodily femininity—she is, medically speaking, a neuter.

As puberty approaches, the ovaries awaken. Little by little, they secrete small doses of estrogen into the bloodstream. The estrogen in the blood acts as a chemical messenger, alerting cells throughout the body that the neuter girl must now turn into a woman. The breasts swell, the uterus enlarges, pubic and axillary hair grows, and the entire body takes on softer contours. At last, the ovary releases its first egg. Shortly afterwards, the first menstrual period occurs—the event that marks the child's transformation into a woman.

The ovaries, awakened to their regular monthly tour of duty, are now pouring larger quantities of estrogen into the bloodstream. Measured by chemical analysis, the total amount of estrogen seems quite small. For example, the daily output of estradiol—the most prominent type among the various estrogens—is no more than about the equivalent of one-thousandth of a grain of sugar. Yet so powerful is the substance that even this tiny amount is enough to change a girl into a woman.

At the end of adolescence, she is at last complete. Everything about her is designed to attract the male, and she becomes increasingly aware of her power. Her personality changes accordingly, as does her entire view of the world. It is indeed fascinating to consider how a chemical substance such as estrogen shapes the spirit and defines the purpose of a human being.

The social implications of these physical changes set the pattern of the woman's life. Her bodily competence as a woman—in addition to the emotional changes engendered by her bodily development—gives her the right to marry, to procreate, and to wield continuing influence in the lives of her husband and children.

The key to this development again lies in the double life of the ovaries, acting both as repositories for eggs and as endocrine glands producing hormones. Endocrine glands pour their secretion into the blood, in contrast to other glands—such as the saliva glands or the tear glands—whose products flow to some body surface, such as the lining of the mouth or the covering of the eye.

Endocrine glands, as we have noted, are chemical factories, producing substances that assure the proper functioning of the body as a whole. The thyroid gland in the throat, for example, governs the rate of metabolism, i.e., the speed with which the body burns up energy. If it is too active, the results are chronic restlessness, agitation, underweight. If it is sluggish, the results are lethargy, sleepiness, lack of ambition, and obesity.

Another important endocrine gland, the pancreas, produces insulin, the substance that controls the amount of sugar in the blood. Too little sugar produces sudden weakness, loss of consciousness, and possibly mental aberrations. Too much sugar results in sluggish reactions, an accumulation of poisons in the cells, and frequently the onset of gangrene.

The adrenal glands, located just above the kidneys, mobilize the body and give it extra strength in moments of stress and danger. They are responsible for the almost-incredible feats accomplished in moments of crisis. They also provide cortisone, which counteracts many of the degenerative processes in the body.

The male gonads (endocrine glands producing sex hormones) make a man grow whiskers, toughen his muscle tissue, and deepen his voice.

As for the female sex glands, the ovaries, they differ from all the other endocrines in several important respects. They switch every month from one product to another: estrogen during the first half of the menstrual cycle, progesterone during the second half. However, as chemical factories they wear out too fast. Halfway in a woman's life, these factories break down—causing the onset of menopause.

Fortunately, we now have a remedy against the untimely shutdown of the ovarian factory. If the ovaries can no longer make estrogen, we can now supply it in the form of tablets. The body doesn't care whether the estrogen on which it thrives is "homegrown" in its own ovaries or imported from the nearest drugstore. Just as long as there's enough of it.

If all the endocrine glands were pouring out their secretions at random, without some kind of central control to assure coordination among all those hormones, the result would be chaos. That is why the entire endocrine system of the body is arranged like a tightly organized corporation in which everybody takes orders from headquarters.

Headquarters is literally in the head. At the base of

the brain, in the most inaccessible spot of the entire body, the master gland is cradled in the base of the skull. Known as the pituitary gland, this central station of the endocrine system sends out chemical commands that keep the other glands in various parts of the body working as a team. Then again the pituitary receives chemical "feedback" signals through the blood, telling the master gland how well its commands have been obeyed. In this way, the pituitary maintains the proper *balance* between all the various hormones in the bloodstream.

It is from this master gland that the ovary receives a special chemical each month (a follicle stimulating hormone—F.S.H.) which causes a number of follicles to mature. This results in the production of increasing and adequate amounts of estrogen as the readying of the egg proceeds. As soon as the pituitary senses the sharp rise of estrogen in the blood, it "knows" that its orders have been followed. It then sends out the next chemical command to the ovaries: "Prepare the corpus luteum and make progesterone to build up the uterine lining for the reception of the embryo." This order is transmitted from the head to the ovaries through a chemical (a luteinizing hormone—L.H.) which triggers ovulation. After the uterine lining breaks down during menstruation, the pituitary gives the signal to start all over.

You can see how this complicated central chemical command station of the entire body can be thrown into turmoil during menopause. Ovaries that no longer produce eggs no longer secrete estrogen. The master gland—the pituitary—senses the lack of estrogen. Frantically it sends out more follicle-stimulating hormone, saying in effect: "Step Up Estrogen Production —Fast!" But the dying ovaries no longer respond. Like a frustrated field commander, repeating orders to lost troops, the pituitary churns out more demands for estrogen. As a result of this futile attempt, the pituitary itself becomes unbalanced, upsetting all the other endocrine glands in the body. If headquarters is in turmoil, confusion soon invades the ranks. The body's entire chemical system goes haywire, producing many of the distressing and dangerous menopausal symptoms.

Because the pituitary gland is located in such a central position in the brain, pituitary secretions flood the adjacent hypothalamus, the brain center which controls many vital life processes. The nerves emanating from the hypothalamus, known as the autonomic nervous system, regulate such activities as breathing, intestinal movement, heart action, the contraction and expansion of arteries, and the enlargement of the pupils of the eyes. As the focal point of this autonomic nervous system, the hypothalamus has been called "a brain within the brain". It is the point at which our conscious thoughts and feelings touch upon the unconscious automatic functions of the body; those over which we have no voluntary control.

Through this link between the pituitary—representing the endocrine system—and the nervous system, the entire body becomes involved in emotional responses. The gasp of horror, the breath held in suspense, the pupil enlarging in surprise, the flush of embarrassment, the sweat of anxiety, and the heart pounding in fear—all these are evidence of this mind-body link.

The same mechanism also produces permanent bodily effects from emotional causes. Nervous tension, by acting on the hypothalamus, can produce digestive disorders, including gastric and duodenal ulcers, diarrhea, and colitis. It may interfere with the functions of the liver, pancreas, and kidney, causing dangerous accumulations of toxic substances in the body. Bladder functions can be similarly affected by emotional disorders.

Again the link to menopause becomes apparent. The hypothalamus—the control center of the autonomic nervous system—takes a terrific buffeting when the pituitary gland reacts to the stoppage of estrogen production in the ovaries. The hypothalamus, in turn, sends out alarms throughout the autonomic nervous system with unpredictable emotional results. The hectic and disorganized messages reach the heart, the liver, the intestines, the colon, and other parts of the body. These organs, previously so well controlled by the hypothalamus, now revolt against the menopausal confusion. In their own way, the organs protest against the panic in the central command. The net result is that the post-menopausal woman suffers a decline in *all* of her bodily functons—not merely in those connected with reproduction. Such perturbation of the body indeed puts her mind and spirit to a grueling test, and it is hardly surprising that many women become mentally disturbed in their menopausal years.

Let me, however, call attention once more to the sequence of these events: it is the physical disturbance that causes the mental upset—not the other way around. The treatment of menopausal disorders must therefore begin with correcting the physical situation. In most cases, the mental situation will then take care of itself. Once these causal relations are understood, it seems folly indeed to treat menopause as "a state of mind" and ignore its physical causes.

To summarize the role of estrogen in the pituitary control center in the brain, I should like to quote a simile I once heard at a popular medical lecture. The speaker compared the pituitary to an irascible man who controls his entire family with strict discipline. But if something goes wrong, he is likely to fly into a rage and smash up the whole house. Estrogen, on the other hand, is like a calm, tactful woman who smoothes his irascible temper and keeps him from going to extremes. As long as estrogen is on hand, the temperamental pituitary keeps calm order in the endocrine family. But when estrogen is absent the overwrought pituitary makes a shambles of the entire household of the body.

The pituitary gland is by no means the only part of the body that eagerly welcomes the ministrations of estrogen. Almost any cell in a woman's body becomes stronger and more capable of doing its job when it is nourished by an adequate supply of estrogen. For example, take the effect of estrogen on the most distantly outlying of all body cells—the skin.

There is hardly anything lovelier to sight and touch than the skin of a young woman of about twenty—so smooth, pliant, and delicate. Again it is estrogen which may claim the main credit for this loveliness.

In the early stages of puberty, the skin is often marred by acne—a condition that brings much unhappiness to young girls. This is usually a sign that the ovaries are not yet producing their full quota of estrogen. Once a girl matures into young adulthood and the ovaries become more proficient at their task, the acne usually clears up spontaneously.

However, in some cases, no spontaneous recovery occurs. I recall the case of a young nurse whose face was covered with purulent acne. This completely robbed her of self-confidence. She slithered in and out of rooms, as if to hide from sight. Nobody paid her any attention, and in a patronizing sort of way, I began to feel sorry for her. One day I surprised myself by taking her brusquely by the arm and asking her: "Would you like to be a beautiful girl?"

The question was as inane as it was tactless. I had said it entirely on impulse. Tears filled the girl's eyes.

Uncomfortable about having embarrassed her, I asked her to come to my office. A test revealed that her estrogen secretion rate was extremely low. I prescribed estrogen injections (1.66 milligrams estradiol benzoate weekly for the first three weeks of her menstrual cycle) along with vitamin A and hydrochloric acid capsules. Improvement was slow, but two years later her face was clear and astoundingly pretty. Even more remarkable was the change in her attitude toward life. She is now married and has had her third child. I never see her any more, but every Christmas she sends me a bottle of whiskey. Once a note was attached: "God made you notice me: Wednesday, March 8, 1949, at 6:10 p.m."

After menopause the skin again reacts to the absence of estrogen and becomes dry and wrinkled. While estrogen therapy cannot restore the magic bloom of youth to the skin of a middle-aged woman, it will often make the skin smooth, supple, and taut again. In addition to estrogen taken in the form of tablets, the skin may be refreshed by estrogen-containing creams and ointments available through a doctor's prescription.

Estrogen also determines to a considerable degree the development of a woman's breasts. Probably no other part of a woman's anatomy is as directly related to her self-confidence as a woman. One reason why our culture—particularly in the United States—attaches such importance to the female bosom lies in the development of modern media of mass communication. Magazine editors, advertisers, TV directors, and moviemakers—the men who make the cultural climate— quickly learned the elementary lesson that to show the female figure in some unnaturally dramatized fashion is a surefire way to rivet male attention. The trend began about half a century ago when it first became feasible to reproduce photographs in print. This gave rise to the concept of the "cover girl," which grew into the concept of "glamour" and later degenerated into a kind of mammary cult.

With all these spurious, commercial values attached to the shape and size of breasts, it is hardly surprising that a woman is rarely satisfied with her natural endowments. She is unhappy if her breasts are too small; self-conscious if they are too large. Advertisers bombard her with urgent advice about the shape and construction of brassieres, the efficacy of breast-growing creams (often fraudulent and dangerous). Some women are driven by these irrational pressures to have their breasts surgically altered or inflated with paraffin —a doubtful step whose psychological benefits do not always justify such drastic medical procedure.

Worrying about her breasts often causes a woman to develop a pathological fear of cancer, despite the fact that only six percent of all women develop such malignancies.

Before discussing the physical structure of the breasts and the effect of estrogen on their development, we should briefly comment on the social aspects of this part of a woman's body. Quite aside from their biological functions, a woman's breasts are—if we may coin such an expression—a psychological organ. This is true not only in our particular breast-conscious society, but has been so in other cultures at all times—a fact evidenced by such customs as painting a woman's exposed breasts with ornamental patterns among certain primitive tribes. My clinical interviews with countless women have convinced me that the breasts are closely linked in a woman's mind to her innermost, private self. They are part of her psyche. It is my impression that too many doctors—particularly surgeons —are not sufficiently aware of these psychological implications and conduct breast examinations without proper regard for the emotional factors involved. Also, they are sometimes too hasty in recommending surgical removal of a breast, not taking into account the mental anguish such an operation entails.

It might make a woman less breast-conscious to realize that, for any normal man, breasts are by no means a woman's principal attraction.

Roving about at a party, a footloose male might scan his surroundings at floor level, searching for a pair of trim legs. A slow upward sweep of the eyes thereupon assesses the general posture of his object of interest. As a physician professionally trained in the art of observation, it has not escaped me that what turns male heads at a gathering is not a woman's face or even her figure. It is an erect, graceful posture that invariably commands attention. Men are generally unaware that it was a woman's stance that drew their notice. If asked what focused their attention on that particular woman, they would not be able to define posture as the decisive factor.

Once his interest is aroused, a man usually takes a

rather systematic inventory of a woman's appearance. He assesses her face, though beauty in the classic sense does not seem to rank high as a sexual attractant; then he examines her manner of dress, reacting strongly to that indefinable quality of chic (which, by the way, has little to do with being merely fashionable—there are women who look more chic in dungarees than others do in Dior). The critical survey then proceeds to her hands, teeth, and throat. By that time the investigating male is doubtlessly edging closer in order to sample her voice and manner of speech. Eventually, his eyes limn the contour of her breasts. But this mammary survey, in most social situations, has low priority. I wish more women would realize this. It may ease their breast-centered anxieties.

Excessively large breasts do not seem to trouble most women, although I know of cases where surgical reduction of the mammaries was requested by the patient and successfully carried out. Small breasts, by contrast, are often a source of unhappiness to young women, except in times when flat-chestedness is fashionable. If the smallness of the breast is an inherited characteristic, there is little that can be done except injection with paraffin. Quite frequently, however, small breasts are a symptom of over-all sexual under-development due to inadequate estrogen level. In those cases, estrogen therapy supplemented by progesterone will slightly increase the size of the breasts, make them firmer, and at the same time increase their erotic sensitivity. The sex hormones will also lead to fuller development of the genitals.

A typical patient of this kind came to me when she was thirty-two years of age. Because of her sexual underdevelopment she had not had many suitors before. Recently, however, a man had become seriously interested in her. She was desperate when she consulted me. "He cannot marry me as I am," she wailed. After a few months of estrogen and progesterone therapy, her breasts had nicely filled out and her genitals no longer presented an obstacle to marriage.

The form of the breast is mostly a matter of inheritance, but estrogen and progesterone can influence the shape. Estrogen develops the duct system within the breast that produces and gathers the milk; progesterone chiefly affects the surrounding tissue. Together, in correct proportion, the two hormones assure full mammary growth and balanced form.

Hormone-deficient breasts respond beautifully to treatment in as little as three to four months. After six months the breasts reach the fullest development possible, given the patient's particular heredity. But it is not merely size alone that gratifies young women so treated. There is also a new firmness in her breasts and a new tactile sensitivity at certain times of the month.

I emphasize again that this treatment is effective only if the cause of mammary underdevelopment is low estrogen level. Before a woman embarks on such therapy, her estrogen level must be determined by test. If the young woman has her full quota of estrogen, added hormone therapy will not increase breast size. It would be a waste of time and money and might possibly lead to unwanted side effects.

Similarly futile, in my experience, is treatment of the breasts with hormone creams and ointments. Hormones given by mouth are invariably more effective.

After menopause, when estrogen and progesterone sink to a low level, the breasts begin to shrivel and sag. Once the supply of those two nourishing hormones is cut off, the breasts become pendulous, wrinkled, and flabby. Often the skin of the breasts coarsens and is covered with scales. The breasts lose their erotic sensitivity and sometimes do not even respond to pain stimuli. Only timely estrogen replacement therapy can prevent this premature decline of a woman's symbol of femininity.

The womb exhibits a similar dependence on estrogen. At puberty, when estrogen arrives in increasing quantities, the cells of a young girl's tiny uterus literally wallow in it, engorging themselves on the growth-stimulating hormone and enlarging the uterus to its full size and strength.

During pregnancy, the uterus expands to enormous size to hold anywhere from one to five babies, plus the surrounding fluid and the nourishing placenta. Its tissues are drenched in estrogen, which is at that time produced in the placenta as well as in the ovaries. A pregnant woman has an estrogen level up to 600 times greater than that of a non-pregnant woman. After reaching a certain maximal value, the estrogen concentration drops sharply, thereby giving the signal for the onset of labor and stimulating the immensely powerful contractions of the uterus which expel the baby through the narrow and often unyielding birth passage. The pressure exerted in this act of birth is at least eighty pounds per square inch—a truly astonishing feat of sheer muscular strength.

In my opinion, a woman having experienced several pregnancies is basically healthier, more infection-resistant, and more feminine than her barren sisters. During her period of gestation, every cell in her body, from head to toe, becomes suffused with an abundance of age-retarding estrogen that otherwise would not have been produced.

Today, of course, there is no longer any need to become pregnant just to have enough estrogen in the body. Any desired amount can be taken in the form of tablets. Still, I seem to detect a certain look or attitude in some women that I might call "the birth-control look." Women who have plenty of sex but no children somehow strike me as vaguely tense and unfulfilled. But it may be that mere sentiment beclouds my observation.

The only function of the uterus is to furnish a temporary home for the unborn child. It does not enter into a woman's organic or sexual functioning in any way. Yet, as many women know, it is frequently a starting point for cancer. When diseased, it may be advisable to remove the uterus by an operation known as hysterectomy. A section in Chapter 6 will discuss this type of surgery in relation to estrogen therapy and continued femininity.

Estrogen interacts closely with the Fallopian tubes

that connect the uterus to the ovaries. It causes the tubes to widen and stimulates the little fibers in the tubes that push along the egg.

As for the vagina, estrogen causes a truly remarkable transformation. A young girl's frail and fragile tract expands under the influence of pubertal estrogen. Its lining thickens and darkens, becomes resistant to infection and populated with beneficial germs that keep the bad germs from multiplying. It becomes extremely elastic so that even an unusually thick penis can be admitted. Estrogen provides the vagina with such strength, durability, and elasticity that even the baby's relatively enormous head may pass through it without lasting damage to the mother.

The abundance of estrogen in late adolescence accounts for the fact that a girl of fifteen to twenty suffers less vaginal damage in childbirth than a woman of thirty-five to forty, whose estrogen supply is beginning to wane as she approaches menopause. In pregnancies after the age of thirty-five, an effort should be made to keep the baby reasonably small at the time of birth (about 6½ pounds) so as to minimize overstretching of the vagina and other pelvic complications.

Few processes in the entire body are as dramatic as the estrogenic transformation of the vagina. However, since it occurs in what are, quite literally, a woman's private parts, this amazing physiological event is rarely noticed.

All the more reason for the woman's pained distress

when, after menopause, the lack of estrogen causes the vagina to revert to its previous brittle and inelastic condition. Indeed, vaginal irritation, inflammation, and sexual inadequacy is one of the most embarrassing symptoms of menopause to a woman whose spirit is still willing. What untold misery and frustration could be alleviated in this respect alone if the benefits of estrogen therapy were more widely known!

Quite aside from its specific effects on the breasts and genitals, estrogen plays an important part in the total conformation of the female body. We have already noted its effect on the skin—the body's outermost cells. The structure of the bones is also subject to the influence of estrogen. For instance, the absence of estrogen in childhood permits the bones to grow and lengthen. But at the age of puberty, the new outpouring of estrogen gradually inhibits this growth. Without this estrogen action on the bones, a girl would become a gaunt, gawky, ill-proportioned creature.

A woman's pelvis spreads out broadly at the hips—in contrast to a man's slimmer and more vertical hip structure. This difference, too, is imparted to the growing cells through estrogen—the hormone of femininity. Some estrogen-poor women do not develop a sufficiently wide pelvic structure and develop narrow, boyish hips. Such women frequently suffer difficult childbirth.

Estrogen is also involved in keeping the tissues supple and moist, which makes for healthy gums and resistance to infection in the conjunctiva of the eyes.

Most important, estrogen helps assure the flexibility of joints. When we marvel at a young woman's litheness it seems tragic to think that all too soon such a woman may lose her beguiling grace simply because she fails to keep up her estrogen balance.

The reason for the pervasive influence of estrogen is that it affects every single cell of the female body from the little toe all the way to the top of the head. This over-all, controlling power stems from the role of estrogen in the basic energy household of the body.

Protein, the basic substance of all cells, contains nitrogen as one of its most important ingredients. Estrogen enables the cells to assimilate nitrogen more efficiently from food.

This gives rise to the concept of the nitrogen balance. It works just like your bank balance. If more nitrogen goes into the body than is taken out through waste products, you have a positive nitrogen balance and are ahead. But if you deplete your nitrogen "bank account" and spend more than you get, you wind up with a negative nitrogen balance. The result, invariably, is bankruptcy of your health.

Even if you go on a high-protein diet, you cannot make up this loss if estrogen is lacking in your system. The cells simply refuse to assimilate nitrogen from the protein in your food.

The importance of estrogen for proper nitrogen utilization has been recognized by pediatricians for some time. If a young girl is weak, sickly, and frail, and fails to gain weight, estrogen is often given to the child for a limited time despite the risk of premature (though temporary) feminization. (Androgen is given to boys in this condition.) The results are astounding. In a matter of days, pallor disappears, the child rapidly gains weight and becomes noticeably stronger and more vigorous.

Similarly, old people with a wasting illness are treated with sex hormones to build up their nitrogen balance and assure proper nutrition of their cells.

Again the implication for menopause is apparent. As the estrogen level declines in post-menopausal years, cells throughout the body lose their ability to utilize nitrogen efficiently. The first visible signs occur in the muscles. Arms and legs loose their suppleness and strength, becoming gaunt and stringy. The neck grows scrawny; grace and rhythm of movement soon depart along with proper muscular coordination. Even physicians rarely realize that the characteristic ungainliness of older women is not so much a matter of stiff joints— although they, too, are involved—but is caused chiefly by the nitrogen starvation of muscles and ligaments.

The same kind of tissue starvation due to negative nitrogen balance also occurs in the internal organs of post-menopausal women. The heart, the stomach and intestines, the smooth muscles of the major arteries, the bronchial tubes, the bladder and kidneys—all become damaged in some degree. At a later point, we shall discuss in greater detail the relation of estrogen to heart disease, coronary attacks, and strokes. For the present, I should like to emphasize the general nature of these changes spreading through the entire body. This explains why menopause is so difficult to define as a specific disease yet can produce truly catastrophic conditions for the whole organism.

The first signs of disturbance usually come from the digestive tract. At a certain point in life you suddenly notice that you can no longer eat everything you like. Food lies heavily in your stomach, gas rolls around your intestines. Soon after you notice that your heart pounds harder after you climb the stairs. It no longer gets any cooperation from the arteries, whose muscles have gone on strike for more nitrogen. Your blood pressure no longer rises and falls in normal response to exercise, rest, and emotion. It becomes elevated and static as the result of arterial stiffening.

When you visit your doctor, complaining of these symptoms, he may give you a laxative for your constipation, and all kinds of pills for your sciatica, gout, or whatever he calls it. Chances are he won't give you estrogen, not considering that the single cause of all your distress might really be an estrogen deficiency resulting from menopause.

All the symptoms we have described here might eventually result from age alone. But there is no reason why they should be allowed to vex any woman younger than seventy-five. The key to the total syndrome, as we have seen, is estrogen deficiency. Now at last—thanks to the achievements of modern pharmaceutical science—this condition is wholly preventable and curable by replacement therapy with estrogen tablets.

How, then, do you know whether or not you are estrogen deficient? Fortunately, you need not wait for any symptoms to develop. It is possible to determine your estrogen level by a very simple, brief, and totally painless test described in detail in Chapter 6. In effect this test provides an index of your femininity. It takes only a few minutes at your doctor's office, but the test will reveal the vital clue from which you can plot your future as a woman. Your body's health and your soul's contentment may hinge on just that one decision: to have your estrogen level checked.

5

Menopause—The Loss of Womanhood and the Loss of Good Health

AT THE RISK of seeming paradoxical, I should like to launch into the subject of menopause by discussing its effect on men. Menopause covers such a wide range of physical and emotional symptoms that the implications are by no means confined to the woman. Her husband, her family, and her entire relationship to the outside world are affected almost as strongly as her own body. Only in this broader context can the problem of menopause—as well as the benefits of a hormonal cure—be properly appreciated.

A melodramatic and, in retrospect, amusing incident that occurred in my own practice many years ago illuminates the intensity of some husbands' feelings about their wives' menopause.

It was quite late in the evening, toward the end of my consulting hours, when my receptionist told me there was a man in the waiting room who wished to see me. Male patients being a rarity in a gynecologist's practice, I agreed to talk to him, even though he had come without appointment.

A skinny man in his fifties with a sharp and sallow face slid rather furtively through the door. His manner was an unpleasant mixture of embarrassment and aggressiveness. For a while he just fidgeted.

"Doc," he finally blurted out, "they tell me you can fix women when they get old and crabby."

I sidestepped the implied question and let him tell more of his story: "She's driving me nuts. She won't fix meals. She lets me get no sleep. She picks on me all the time. She makes up lies about me. She hits the bottle all day. And we used to be happily married.

"She's been to three doctors already," he continued. "They all tell her it's 'the change' and nothing can be done about it. Now she tells me to get out and never come back. But I won't. It's *my* home. And if anyone's going, she is."

He reached into his back pocket—in those days shoulder holsters were still unknown—and quietly laid a .32 automatic on the edge of my desk.

"If you don't cure her, I'll kill her."

I looked at him doubtfully. "You think that would be better for you?" I asked cautiously, my mind reeling with all I had heard about armed madmen in doctors' offices. But I was wrong. The man was completely rational.

"I got advanced T.B.," my visitor explained. "I was X-rayed again just last week. My doctor tells me that I have less than a year to live. I want to die in peace— and I can't if she's around."

My client, I later discovered, was a prominent member of the Brooklyn underworld. The proposed method of dealing with his wife apparently seemed to him quite proper and businesslike. Fortunately no calamity occurred. I accepted his wife as a patient and she responded well to intensive twice-a-week estrogen injections. Her disposition improved noticeably after three weeks, and soon she was very busy taking care of her sick husband.

I heard no more from him directly. He died on schedule and I received an invitation to his elaborate funeral. His widow felt genuine grief at his death.

Despite the fact that the years have added comic overtones to this episode, I have often been haunted by the thought that—except for the tiny stream of estrogen which I passed into her body through the hypodermic needle—this woman might have died a violent death at the hands of her own husband. Thanks to the healing power of the estrogen I administered, there had been an opportunity for reconciliation. I was deeply touched when she told me some time afterward that she had been able to instill in her husband during the last weeks of his life a sense of repentance and of religious hope for the salvation of his otherwise-lost soul.

Outright murder may be a relatively rare consequence of menopause—though not as rare as most of us might suppose. Yet the psychological equivalent of murder in the form of broken family relations and hatred between husband and wife is a common result of menopausal change. Medical statistics can never convey the staggering total of sheer misery inflicted upon such families by menopausal side-effects.

These mental changes totally alter a woman's position in relation to her family, her community, and—most important—herself. This condition in itself represents an overwhelming crisis in a woman's life. Only a little more than a decade ago, an English woman physician, the late Dr. J. Malleson pinpointed a certain type of emotional disturbance typical of many women in their middle years and coined the term "menopausal negativism" for this common aberration. Until Dr. Malleson's pioneer study in this field was published in the British medical journal *Lancet* in 1953, the medical profession had generally closed its eyes to this vast area of human suffering.

The degree of mental disturbance varies widely with different persons. In some women it may manifest itself merely as slight absent-mindedness or irritability. In others, it may grow into a neurosis so severe as to make normal personal adjustments impossible. Many women endure the passing years with cow-like passivity and disinterest; and a disturbingly high number take refuge in alcohol, sleeping pills, and sometimes even in suicide.

We do not yet know precisely what determines the degree of mental disturbance associated with menopause. My own observation is that the quality of a woman's marriage is probably one of the most important factors.

In our civilization, a woman's romantic expectations

during her younger years are seldom fully satisfied by the actualities of her life. Often her choice of a husband was based on a compromise in which her hopes and ideals had to yield to other considerations. With our social pressures toward marriage, a man's mere availability often decides the choice for a girl. Later such women go through their married life subconsciously telling themselves that they might still find fulfillment in love—that the man they had hoped to meet might yet somehow come along.

Such women may make good wives and mothers. They often have great competence and energy in all they undertake, and frequently are successful in business careers. A secret hope—unrealized by themselves —motivates them: "It could happen. He might appear tomorrow, or next year." There may be periods of restlessness in such a woman's life that send her running for comfort to her doctor, her clergyman, or maybe her lawyer. But these anxieties pass. For that indomitable feminine hope within her gives her the will and the strength to live, to struggle, to feel joy, and to suffer and persist.

If such a woman could age gradually and gracefully, like a healthy male, this subconscious hope of personal fulfillment would continue and sustain her until late in life. But nature plays a trick on her. During her best years, she encounters menopause—the end of her womanhood.

To be suddenly desexed is to her a staggering catastrophe that strikes directly at those hidden—and perfectly normal—hopes and motivations that have supported her all along.

Had she been conscious of these femine longings for the kind of sensual and emotional fulfillment that her marriage failed to provide, she could rationally cope with her disappointment and perhaps even accept menopause as the end of these hopes. But since her hope and motivations are mostly unconscious, she is incapable of rationally perceiving her own situation. She only knows dimly that the driving power of her existence has somehow failed her. She thrashes about wildly, often venting a special vindictiveness upon her husband and family. Eventually she subsides into an uneasy apathy that is indeed a form of death within life.

The transformation, within a few years, of a formerly pleasant, energetic woman into a dull-minded but sharp-tongued caricature of her former self is one of the saddest of human spectacles. The suffering is not hers alone—it involves her entire family, her business associates, her neighborhood storekeepers, and all others with whom she comes into contact. Multiplied by millions, she is a focus of bitterness and discontent in the whole fabric of our civilization. And the supreme tragedy is that, in the light of present medical possibilities, all this is unnecessary.

It has been my observation, based on more than forty years of gynecological practice, that women who at some time were genuinely and profoundly in love with their husbands do not develop such extremes of menopausal negativism. This lucky minority—about 20 percent of the patients I have encountered—apparently feel that they have already fulfilled their womanly destinies. One of these women once told me, "If I die tomorrow, I have had all a woman can ever hope for—true love."

Such a woman may regret the loss of her femininity. But unlike those who remained emotionally unfulfilled, she tries to spare her husband her sense of loss and, sublimating her own distress, becomes particularly considerate of her husband and family. Her physical ordeal does not alter her basic disposition, and the sadness she feels at the waning of her womanhood she usually keeps to herself. Of course, she is no less aware than any other woman of the physical changes that accompany menopause, and encounters with a mirror that reveal the decline of her body at this stage of life are no less painful to her than to other women.

I have also noticed that such women—the lucky ones who have known deeper dimensions of love—are usually the most eager to begin estrogen therapy when told of this possibility. The happy woman more quickly leaps at the chance to prolong her normal, healthy endowment of femininity.

As a physician, however, I was reminded every single day of my practice that these happy women are exceptions. My main concern has been with the approximately eighty percent of women who have never been overwhelmingly in love. I have tried to help them retain a physical basis for that seemingly essential hope of feminine fulfillment.

In addition to the experience of love, or the lack of it, the severity of menopausal negativism depends on several other factors. Social status, education, native intelligence, and vocational achievement usually exert a strong influence.

Women with ample financial means and secure social standing generally manage to conceal whatever private dismay they feel at this stage of life. With travel, cultural activities, and social diversions open to them, they rarely accept the fading of their womanhood with passive resignation. Actresses, and career women, accustomed to exercise control over their conditions, fight back at fate. Cosmetics and corsetry are their usual weapons. Husbands are usually discarded at this stage, and a series of lovers become busily engaged in playing their part in a costly charade designed to provide the woman with an illusion of continued femininity. While such women escape the more passive forms of menopausal negativism, their obsessive and futile response to physical reality can bring them nothing but unhappiness.

Anyone who has ever been employed in a business directed by a menopausal woman executive is familiar with another variant of this syndrome. The work week becomes a futile, inefficient round of violent ups and downs, adult tantrums, and pointless chicanery. The woman in a position of authority has a ready-made means of side-stepping the passive kind of menopausal negativism. She is presented with an irresistible and unlimited opportunity to take out her frustrations on her employees.

It should be pointed out that the problem here is not merely one of "bitchiness"—a trait by no means confined to women of a certain age or condition. The menopausal syndrome is based on an erratic disorientation of the woman's entire frame of mind, a combination of fixed ideas and unpredictable caprice. In a business situation, this plays havoc not merely with the morale of the woman's subordinates, but it may also lead to serious errors of executive judgement. With more and more women entrusted with decision-making posts in business, government, and in various institutions, the effects of menopause present a new type of management problem that has yet to be fully understood by the experts of corporate administration—all the more so since the syndrome develops at a time when businesswomen are at the apex of their careers and have attained their greatest range of responsibility and power.

In contrast to celebrities or women in the business world, the typical upper-middle-class housewife lacks the opportunities to externalize her menopausal problems. In the usual suburban environment of such well-to-do families, women often resort to quieter, more melancholic forms of self-deception. They pathetically pretend to themselves that they had been truly in love—back when there had still been time.

Not that the marriage of such a woman had been necessarily unhappy. The marriage ceremony had thrilled everybody in the family. They were such a nice couple. In bed, the young bride tried hard to persuade herself that her husband was handsome and gallant. While this wasn't quite satisfactory at first, sex had become distinctly enjoyable to her over the years. The family's financial struggle, the children, and the building of a home had bound her close to her husband through shared experience. And Bill was such a good man. And successful in his business. So she didn't really mind that he was a little too heavy, always tired, and that he drank too much at times.

It might have helped if he had made a few decisions himself occasionally instead of leaving so many responsibilities to her. She knew he could take command in a crisis, but normally he all but ignored his role as head of the house. He preferred to have her assume this prerogative. Once she had welcomed this and been proud of his trust. But now she was bored by it all. She analyzed her plight in terms of a time-honored cliché! If only once he had been angry—grabbed her and shaken her—shown her who was master—and then taken her in his embrace and crushed the breath out of her . . . But now it was too late. . . .

I have known many cases where such women in their forties, after years of seemingly happy marriage, would turn to the grocery boy or the gardener for one last fling, or—if no such men were available—would go prospecting in local bars.

Contrary to the popular image, many such women

are in no way slovenly. Characteristically, they are still attractive and would have done far better to search for adventure within their own social circle among men capable of appreciating their qualities and charm. But panicked by the first signs of menopause, they desperately throw themselves at any man in whose eyes they may find quick acknowledgement of a more elemental appeal. They vainly seek to recapture the fresh and generous allure that was theirs when they were young and that, they imagine, was wasted on a prosaic husband. They are racked by a deep nostalgia for something that never had been. In a maze of longing and delusion they sometimes lose touch with reality, and thus a menopausal neurosis develops.

It is on the next lower rung of the social scale that the most pitiful cases of menopausal negativism are usually found. In the vast social and spiritual wasteland below the comfortable suburban strata, in the drabness of the lower middle class, many factors combine to render a woman psychologically helpless. Typically, such a woman, shackled to a dull, commonplace man, lacks that margin of imagination, cultural interest, and developed taste that helps upper-class women to fight back against menopausal despair, no matter how misguided their methods.

For the lower-middle-class woman, the range of available options is sharply curtailed. She has sense enough to know that, in her restrictive environment, a love affair in the casual suburban style is out of the question. She rarely has the inclination—let alone the time—to occupy herself with new interests such as volunteer hospital work, community service, amateur theater groups, and other activities that might help her retain a positive frame of mind. So she gradually sinks into a state of almost bovine passivity.

Such women generally flock together in small groups of three or four. Not that they have anything to share but their boredom and trivial gossip. Clustering together in monotonous gregariousness, they hide themselves from the rest of the world. They go together to the same hairdresser to have their hair tinted purple. As though they were schoolgirls again, they dress alike and buy the same little hats. They hobble slowly to the delicatessen shop to buy day after day the same cold roast beef and potato salad, for they have long ago resigned from the more challenging responsibilities of their kitchens.

Typically such women have no trace of humor. Spontaneous laughter is unknown to them, though they are capable of a kind of malicious cackle. Their negativism becomes so deeply engrained that often they barely notice what goes on about them. Unseeing, unfeeling, they stumble through the years that could have been filled to the brim with life's most positive values.

This picture is by no means overdrawn. Strolling through any drab neighborhood on a sunny afternoon, you can see such women sitting on the stoops of their houses, oblivious to everything—a total loss to themselves and their families.

Whatever its manifestations and in whatever social setting, menopausal negativism can be treated if recognized early enough. It takes a combination of estrogen therapy and psychological aid. The hormone restores the woman physically, but it is also important to revive her sense of values and her level of motivation. The understanding and cooperation of her husband and her family during her psychological recovery most certainly contribute to the success of the estrogen therapy.

Unfortunately, this negativism is not generally considered to be a condition demanding medical help. Too often, it is simply regarded as a natural symptom of aging, and neither family nor physicians are aware of the possibility of effective treatment. This is doubly tragic because, in its advanced state, menopausal negativism no longer responds to treatment and becomes virtually incurable.

It may be reassuring to reflect that any woman reading this book, even if suffering from other menopausal symptoms, is certainly not suffering from an advanced form of menopausal negativism. If she were, she would not be in the least interested in facing the truth about herself. In fact, she probably would not be reading any book at all.

These psychological symptoms of menopause have given rise to the widely-held misconception that the condition of menopause is "all in the head" and that it is primarily a mental problem. This is a flagrant confusion of cause and effect. There is nothing "mental" about menopause except some of its consequences. Its origins are clearly and overwhelmingly physical, and it is high time that this fact be recognized both by the medical profession and the public.

A woman may come to her doctor with definite physical symptoms—hot flashes, dry mucous membranes, disturbed vision, and aching joints. Yet her doctor may tell her that she is just emotionally upset and send her home with a tranquilizer. To my mind this is like telling a person with a broken leg that his trouble—and his pain—is purely imaginary. Yet this blind, irrational view of menopause still persists as the basis of standard medical practice. Enlightened physicians who see menopause for what it is—a preventable and curable deficiency disease—are still in the minority.

Therefore, one must emphasize again and again that, by means of recently developed techniques of hormonal treatment, it is now possible to restore full femininity even to women long past menopause. And if you have not yet entered the menopause or are only a few years beyond childbearing age, you never need suffer any of these symptoms at all. Preventive treatment can eliminate the monopause entirely.

When a woman goes into panic during menopause, she is merely responding to her instincts, which tell her truthfully that the loss of estrogen is for her—as for any woman—a supreme tragedy. She senses, quite literally in her bones, and in every part of her body, that menopause marks the end of her womanhood. The inner dynamo that energizes her entire being has ceased to function. Indeed, her mental distress is a quite natural response to this deep, instinctive knowledge. The task of physicians, at this point in the history of medicine, is to replace a woman's natural terror with the assurance that menopausal suffering is now "obsolete"—that the modern woman may enjoy her womanhood as long as she lives.

6

Feminine Once More and Forever

ABOUT A DECADE ago, my practice included a patient named Elsie G., a lively spinster aged fifty-five at the time. Enjoying a small inherited fortune, she led a pleasantly active life, centered around clubs, community activities, and frequent trips to New York, about an hour's train ride from her pleasant home overlooking the Hudson River. Elsie took an intelligent interest in the management of her investments, and her weekly schedule of committee meetings, theater visits, and social engagements would have taxed the energies of a woman half her age. Yet Elsie somehow managed to sail through her routine with evident enjoyment and gracious aplomb.

Her sister Alice, though sharing the same background, seemed like Elsie's antithesis. Two years younger than Elsie, Alice was nearly always tired, and suffered frequent headaches, sudden sweats, high blood pressure, and an almost chronic state of depression. Her teeth were giving her trouble and she constantly complained of backache so severe that she was partially incapacitated for days at a time. She rarely went out, took no interest in her former activities. This seemed all the more surprising since Alice until a few years earlier had been an inveterate and accomplished golfer and a champion horsewoman. Though she had become severely hypochondriacal and constantly spoke of her many real and imagined ailments, she was generally distrustful of the medical profession. A local doctor—the only one who enjoyed her rather grudging confidence—blamed her backaches on the "thinning of her bones" and ascribed her entire syndrome of multiple complaints to "the change of life." He—and Alice—were content to let it go at that.

Elsie, on the other hand, had been on a regular estrogen routine ever since she had become my patient several years before.

It would be tempting to credit the striking difference between the two women to the benefits of estrogen therapy, without any further thought. Yet other factors might have been responsible, even though the hereditary constitution of the two sisters was evidently similar. I carefully inquired into the possibility of nutritional differences between the two women as well as into their medical histories. From a medical viewpoint, their histories were entirely similar and unremarkable. Until the onset of Alice's difficulties, both had been in consistently good health. Aside from a case of bronchitis and a broken leg (the result of a riding accident), there was nothing of medical interest to report.

The fact that neither of them ever married seemed in some way related to the strong sense of personal independence engendered by their wealth. At any rate, the cause of their spinsterhood was in no way physical.

As for nutrition, both Alice and Elsie, living in the same household, shared the same diet. Both were careful about what they ate—almost to the point of faddism. They were believers in health foods, organic gardening, unsaturated fats, and plenty of vitamins. Their breakfast, for example, regularly included a small array of dietary supplements—a vitamin E capsule, an organic vitamin C capsule, brewer's yeast tablets, a calcium tablet, an iodine tablet, and a vitamin B-complex tablet. These were served up on a small silver tray and solemnly swallowed with skim milk. Granted, this little ceremony of pills at the breakfast table may seem rather effete to the skeptical observer. The point is that, under this sort of regimen, neither of the two sisters was likely to suffer any dietary deficiencies.

Having ruled out obvious discrepancies in nutrition, constitution, hygiene, and environment in this particular situation, it became apparent to me that the two sisters represented a natural test case for the effectiveness of hormone therapy. For the only difference in their dietary routine lay in the little oval yellow tablet which I prescribed for Elsie. Alice had always spurned hormone treatment. Her doctor didn't recommend it, and she herself shared a popular prejudice against it.

"One of these days those pills will give you cancer,"

Alice repeatedly warned her sister. Elsie merely shrugged.

I had discussed the relationship of cancer and estrogen with her and she was fully reassured. But Alice, with her generally anti-medical attitude, refused to consult me and stubbornly clung to her prejudice. Rather than face her problems openly, she querulously sought comfort in her remembered prowess as a sportswoman. From her couch, nursing her backache, she would talk at length of her past accomplishments as a champion golfer. But now, she resigned herself to waiting passively for an improvement of her state of health—for a longed-for tranquility that she naively expected, but which constantly eluded her.

When Elsie first came to me, I had already become convinced as the result of my research in hormone therapy during the 1930's that the entire menopausal syndrome is a preventable disease. And, though several eminent endocrinologists were sympathetic to this view, only a handful of clinical cases had been reported at the time to corroborate the theory. I told Elsie that, if she took her tablet regularly, she would be one of the first women in the history of the human race never to experience the travails of menopause. I anticipated the usual objections—that interfering with nature could only derange the organs and glands, imbue a woman with desires not suitable to her age, and possibly increase the likelihood of cancer—and presented to her some of the arguments outlined in Chapter 8.

I don't believe it was my power of persuasion that

made her accept the proposed estrogen routine. More likely it was her own vitality, her sense of adventure that wouldn't let her miss the chance of being among the first of her species to attain a new destiny, a new biologic freedom that adds health, meaning, and beauty to the life of any woman—wife or spinster.

She was not disappointed, and I remember her gratefully as one of those many courageous woman who put their trust in me at a time when estrogen therapy was still in its early stages. Hundreds of women like Elsie have since helped me develop the simple and reliable clinical procedures that today makes the attainment or restoration of lasting feminity a safe and reliable procedure.

Investigation of the therapeutic uses of estrogens followed close upon Doisy's historic discovery of these hormones in 1923. Curiously, the initial research was carried out largely in agricultural colleges with a hopeful view toward encouraging the sex life of chickens. But it was not long before a number of astute doctors envisioned the newly-discovered hormones as potential benefactors to the human female. The names of the late Dr. Fuller Albright at Harvard Medical School and Dr. Kost Shelton in California are remembered as being among the earliest advocates of the therapeutic use of estrogens.

It was my own good fortune as a young doctor to share in this vital pioneering work. Possibly it was my youthful insouciance that enabled me to persist in a systematic program of clinical trials at a time when most medical opinion was hardened against the very concept of hormone therapy by the obdurate sort of intellectual cement that is compounded equally of prejudice and ignorance.

My therapeutic results in the late twenties were not too encouraging, largely because the pharmaceutical industry had not yet succeeded in refining a sufficiently pure and potent estrogen preparation. My first experiments were carried out with a crude extract made from dried sheep ovaries, whose limited benefits were often outweighed by allergic side effects.

Even in the thirties, when a relatively potent synthetic estrogen—stilbestrol—became available, the side effects remained. Many patients developed nausea, headaches, and skin rashes. Not until a German preparation, estradiol benzoate, was introduced during the late thirties was the problem of side effects finally overcome. At last patients were able to enjoy the benefits of estrogen therapy without concomitant discomfort.

Though estradiol benzoate proved so effective and trouble-free that some clinicians nicknamed it "the Cadillac of hormones," it did not work very well when taken orally. It had to be administered by injection. Since women are notoriously needle-shy, this was a serious disadvantage. Besides, the injections had to be administered by a doctor or nurse, which necessitated frequent visits to the doctor's office—an inconvenience that added considerable to the cost of therapy.

This expensive drawback was finally overcome when the so-called natural conjugated estrogens became available shortly after the outbreak of World War II. The term "conjugated" refers to the chemical linkage of compounds occurring naturally in the living body. Prepared from the urine of mares in whose bodies this chemical linkage is accomplished, conjugated estrogens are now available in convenient tablet form. Thanks to the metabolic refinement resulting from the conjugation process, these preparations are entirely free of side effects.

The introduction of conjugated estrogens in the form of tablets at last opened the way to an eminently practical therapeutic routine which—as shall be explained later—requires no more than two visits per year to the doctor's office.

My own activity in estrogen therapy spans this entire history. In more than forty years of gynecological practice I have administered estrogen to an estimated total of 5,000 women. To the best of my knowledge, my personal work in this area represents by a wide margin the greatest accumulation of clinical data by any single practitioner. Without exception, every case I treated since the introduction of estradiol benzoate showed some degree of improvement. In many cases total avoidance of all menopausal symptoms was achieved, and the percentage of marked amelioration was surprisingly high. In the entire realm of medicine, there are few forms of therapy with a more consistent record of beneficence. In the closing years of my medical career, I take a perhaps pardonable pride in the fact that the sheer bulk of medical statistics drawn from my work seems to augur a widening acceptance of this vital therapy.

At this point in our discussion I can sense my readers urging me to divulge precise and specific details of the treatment that holds such abundant promise for them. Before I can responsibly do so—naming specific medications and dosages—I must point out that such treatment must be supervised by a competent physician and that under no circumstances should you attempt any kind of self-medication. However, if you obtain the cooperation of a physician willing to treat you, there is nothing complicated, nothing difficult, and positively nothing dangerous about the therapy itself. It is not necessary to seek out a specialist. Any medical practitioner can treat you and keep you under the necessary observation. His main qualification, other than general medical competence, should be a genuine interest in your health and happiness; in short, the ability to sympathize with the needs and problems of his patients.

During your first interview with your doctor, he will ask you about your medical history. Be sure you mention any serious illness and operations you may have had. Particularly, you should tell him if there has even been any suspicion of cancer in your case. If you ever had any kidney or liver diseases or thrombophlebitis (blood clots in veins), be sure that your doctor knows about it. Under these special conditions the therapy may have to be modified.

After taking your medical history, your doctor will give you a complete physical examination. He will look especially for enlarged glands, lumps in the breasts, abdominal tumors, pelvic tumors, and similar formations. As you may have guessed, the purpose of this is to discover at an early stage a previously unsuspected cancer. These steps are not taken because of any possible causal connection between hormone treatment and cancer. They are simply a standard procedure in any thorough physical examination. A blood count and urine analysis are also highly advisable.

Some doctors may order specific laboratory tests to determine the amount of various types of hormones excreted in your urine. This is by no means essential, but the decision should be left to your doctor.

An indispensable part of your examination is the so-called Pap Test—short for Papanicolaou, the Greek physician who originated it. It consists of taking a sample of secretion from the vagina and cervix and examining the cells in it under a microscope. This test should be performed in any case twice yearly as a precaution against cancer.

The test itself is very simple and completely painless. Your doctor gently brushes a cotton applicator or spatula against the vaginal wall and cervix to take a sample from the mucous lining. Then he spreads the material he has obtained on a glass slide which, after some preparation, is examined at the laboratory by a cytologist—a cell specialist—under the microscope.

But in addition to this classic Pap Test, your doctor will take another smear from the sides of the upper vagina for a new and different test. When this slide arrives at the laboratory, it is stained with certain dyes. Then, brightly illuminated by the powerful light source of the microscope, it becomes an index of your femininity.

Three different types of body cells are visible on the slide: superficial, intermediate, and parabasal cells. The cytologist in his laboratory makes a careful count of all three cell types. This count answers one of the most crucial questions that ever confront a woman. It tells whether her body is still feminine, or whether it is gradually turning neuter. If eighty percent or more of the total cell counts are superficial cells, you can still rejoice in your full femininity—your body still retains all the qualities that make you a woman. If the count of superficial cells is less than eighty percent, it is a clear warning that your femininity is waning.

But no longer does the cytologist's verdict portend the end of your womanhood. Rather, regard it as a timely cue provided by nature which should prompt immediate countermeasures. Fortunately, the count of your vaginal cells—your "Femininity Index"—provides just such a signal. The proportion of superficial cells in relation to the other two types gives your doctor an accurate indication of the estrogen dosage you

THE FEMININITY INDEX

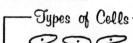

Types of Cells

| Superficial (Mature) | Intermediate (Less Mature) | Parabasal (Immature) |

The Index:

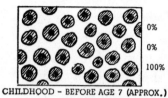

0%	Superficial Cells
0%	Intermediate Cells
100%	Parabasal Cells

 0·0·100

CHILDHOOD - BEFORE AGE 7 (APPROX.)
no estrogen effect

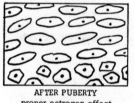

85%	Superficial Cells
15%	Intermediate Cells
0%	Parabasal Cells

85·15·0

AFTER PUBERTY
proper estrogen effect

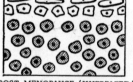

10%	Superficial Cells
20%	Intermediate Cells
70%	Parabasal Cells

10·20·70

POST MENOPAUSE (UNTREATED)
estrogen deficiency

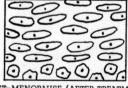

85%	Superficial Cells
15%	Intermediate Cells
0%	Parabasal Cells

85·15·0

POST-MENOPAUSE (AFTER TREATMENT)
proper estrogen effect

require to bring the count back to at least eighty percent.

It is human nature to postpone visits to the doctor. I have friends who would rather endure a toothache than go the dentist. Similarly, I know women who are never at a loss for some "logical" excuse to put off this physical examination. But their logic—if you can call it that—makes even less sense than that of the dentist-shirkers. After all, a dental session may hurt—even though its ultimate object is to stop the pain. Yet a visit to the doctor to take your "Femininity Index" entails no discomfort whatever. Not only that, such a visit signifies hope for every woman.

Many of my patients who came to me regularly twice a year for these tests told me that this routine rewarded them with a wonderful sense of reassurance. They knew that they were the first women in history to benefit from an exact measure of their physical femininity and to have it within their power to maintain—or even to restore—this femininity regardless of age. They came to look upon their visits to the doctor not as an occasion of dread and foreboding. On the contrary: they were events that pointed the way to their self-fulfillment in life—events to be approached not with fear but with eagerness, hope, and exhilaration.

Let us return to your specific case. If you have stopped menstruating, these tests can be made at any time. If you have not yet entered the menopause, the test must be made shortly before probable ovulation—

that is on the eleventh, twelfth, thirteenth, or fourteenth day of the average twenty-eight-day cycle. The
reason for this is that the estrogen level rises and falls
during the menstrual cycle and the vaginal cell count
changes with it. Just before ovulation, the estrogen
level is at its peak.

Taken twice a year, your Femininity Index helps

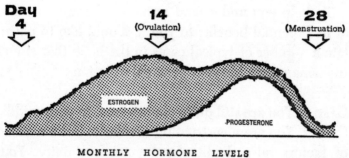

Day **14** **28**
4 (Ovulation) (Menstruation)

ESTROGEN

PROGESTERONE

MONTHLY HORMONE LEVELS
(schematic approximation)

your doctor adjust your estrogen dosage to your body's
demand. Also keep in mind that, since your Femininity
Index measurements are always combined with a Pap
Test, this routine serves as an automatic cancer warning system. If every woman over twenty took this test
twice yearly, cancer of the cervix—one of the most
cruel of all cancers—could be detected early enough
to be cured in nearly every case. In short, the suggested routine not only assures you lasting femininity;
it also betters your chance that you will live to enjoy it
for a long time.

After your initial visit to the doctor, therapy itself is
as simple as taking vitamins. In most cases, all you do

is swallow one tablet a day—except for certain days of the month when you swallow two tablets or none. And you keep this up for the rest of your life.

A variety of estrogen preparations are now available for your doctor to prescribe. Some are natural, some semi-natural, and some synthetic. Personally, I favor natural conjugated estrogens in tablet form. The standard dose is a 1.25-milligram tablet.

To help you understand hormone therapy in terms of its potential benefits to you, I should like to postulate a number of typical cases in the hope that one of them may resemble your personal situation.

CASE 1: You are still quite young—say, in your middle thirties. You are menstruating regularly, but a number of factors raise doubt about your femininity. Your breasts are small, you tend to be frigid. Perhaps you have a tendency to gain weight. Your whole disposition, physical as well as psychological, seems unfeminine. Could your gonads be at fault? Are your ovaries under-active in their hormonal secretion? The answer is quickly gained through the Femininity Index.

Suppose the Femininity Index shows that you are estrogen-deficient. The cure is simple: You take estrogen tablets during the first three weeks of your menstrual cycle. No estrogen is taken during the fourth week.

Depending on your Femininity Index (i.e., the percentage of superficial cells in the vaginal smear), your doctor will prescribe a certain number of tablets to be taken—anywhere from perhaps seven to twenty-one during three weeks of your menstrual cycle. The dosage is calculated to restore your Femininity Index to the normal count of eighty to eighty-five percent superficial cells. Your doctor may suggest repeated Index readings until he establishes the exact number of tablets that will hold your Index constant at the optimum level.

After a relatively short time you will find yourself harmoniously growing into a new state of health, gaining a sense of well-being, developing the positive outlook that results from the knowledge that you have become a person no longer suffering physical impediments to the fulfillment of your feminine role in life.

CASE 2. You are approaching, or have already passed, the age of forty, with perhaps a few menopausal signs and symptoms. Your menstruation is still fairly regular, although decreasing in amount or duration. You are wondering if your body's chemistry is preparing for "The Change." A smear is taken and your Femininity Index shows that the physical basis of your womanhood is indeed in decline.

The therapy under these conditions is precisely the same as for Case 1, the principle being identical in both situations. Physiologically, the estrogen tablets restore the chemical activity of your body to its normal level, allowing you to regain the physical as well as the psychic attributes of womanhood which you would otherwise have lost.

CASE 3. You are a woman in your thirties menstruating irregularly, sometimes skipping a month, or perhaps even two or three months in a row. Possibly there are additional indications of gonadal underactivity, such as small breasts, frigidity, and a tendency to become obese. Following a visit to your doctor, you discover that your Femininity Index shows an estrogen deficiency, which can be cured by taking estrogen tablets from the fifth through the twenty-fourth day of the menstrual cycle. After a while, the doctor will recognize the exact dosage needed to maintain the estrogen level so that your superficial cell count reaches the normal eighty to eighty-five percent. Most often, the dosage turns out to be about twenty estrogen tablets per month.

Yet to restore regularity to your menstrual cycle, something else may be needed in addition to estrogen. You may remember from our previous discussion that the menstrual cycle has two distinct phases—the first part of the cycle being dominated by estrogen, the second part by a progesterone. To induce this natural rhythm of alteration, you may also require a restorative dosage of a progestin.

The reason for progesterone deficiency is that if you do not ovulate no corpus luteum develops. You are thus deprived of your natural source of progesterone.

Fortunately, no specific test is needed to establish

your progesterone level. If you ovulate at all, you have sufficient progesterone. If you fail to ovulate, you are totally deficient. There is no intermediate condition. It further simplifies matters that there is little individual variation in progesterone requirements between one woman and another. The same standard dose, having been previously determined by trial-and-error, nearly always proves satisfactory.

Pure progesterone is not very effective when given by mouth. Progestins, which are chemically related, are preferable. These can be taken orally without loss of potency. One of these—medroxyprogesterone acetate—closely approaches the physiologic effect of progesterone itself. It has proven highly successful in the treatment of progesterone deficiency in irregularly menstruating women.

In addition to the estrogen tablets, your doctor may therefore prescribe half a tablet (five milligrams) of medroxyprogesterone acetate to be taken daily from the fourteenth through the twenty-fourth day of your cycle. You stop taking both estrogen and the progestin after the twenty-fourth day. You may then expect the onset of menstruation on the twenty-seventh or twenty-eighth day. You begin taking estrogen again on the fifth day of the new cycle, counting the first day of bleeding as the beginning of the cycle. Your normal cycle and hormone balance are thus restored.

In some instances this treatment is stopped after six months or a year. Ovulation and the normal menstrual cycle then continue by themselves in natural fashion and may continue for many years, leaving you normally fertile.

CASE 4. You are past forty and have irregular menstrual periods with frequent skipping. You have experienced hot flashes, sudden sweats, nervousness, depression, and other menopausal symptoms. You are sure that The Change has befallen you. Your Femininity Index proves this to be so.

Therapy in this case is identical to that in Case 3. As a result of the treatment, you will regain your full womanhood. But unlike the younger woman in Case 3, the progesterone substitution definitely cannot restore ovulation. You will not become fertile again. But this does not mean that you cannot be fully feminine. Thanks to the treatment outlined here, you can continue the cyclic functions that sustain the health of the entire female body. With estrogen and progestin supplied in the form of tablets, your menstrual cycles can go on indefinitely beyond the time when ovulation ceases.

There is an interesting variant on this routine that may be applied to somewhat younger women who want to obtain birth control along with menopause prevention. If the progestin is taken daily from the fifth through the twenty-fourth day of the cycle simultaneously with estrogen, no ovulation can occur. Hence the woman cannot conceive.

This is a boon for women during the years of approaching menopause. Ovulation at that time of life is irregular and the fertile periods of such women are unpredictable. They may not realize it, but the "rhythm method" of birth control is quite unreliable for them. As a result, many women who may even have believed that they are no longer capable of impregnation find themselves surprised with a so-called "menopause baby." The routine outlined in the foregoing paragraph is a safety measure against such unwanted pregnancies in later life, when birth may be very difficult for the mother. This type of birth control at the same time prevents menopausal symptoms. (There is, in fact, a close relation between hormone therapy and birth control. This will be more fully discussed in Chapter 9.)

CASE 5. You are in your fifties, and almost ten years have gone by since you menstruated for the last time. Your symptoms are those common to many postmenopausal women. You are depressed, chronically fatigued, suffer sleeplessness, a constant ache in the lower back, an itching irritation of the genitals, and perhaps pain during sexual intercourse. Your blood pressure is higher than normal, your breasts have become flabby, and your external genitals have shrunk. All this, you suspect, cannot be part of a natural aging process because your physical decline is happening so fast. Your visit to the doctor and the cell count on your vaginal smear reveal that your Femininity Index has sunk extremely low indeed. You are virtually bankrupt of estrogen.

Your doctor may prescribe one 1.25-milligram estrogen tablet to be taken daily for forty-two days, plus one 10-milligram progestin tablet to be taken daily from the thirty-first through the forty-second day of the treatment. On that day both tablets are discontinued, and two or three days later—as a token of your restored femininity—you will menstruate once again.

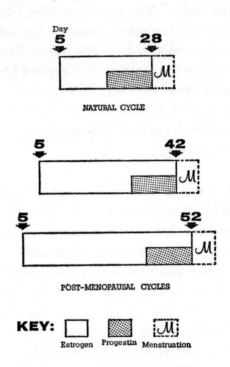

NATURAL CYCLE

POST-MENOPAUSAL CYCLES

KEY: Estrogen Progestin Menstruation

Then you resume taking estrogen tablets on the fifth day of menstruation.

This treatment results in about seven menstruations per year, a cycle of about forty-nine days. After three to five years at that frequency, the treatment can be lengthened to a fifty-two-day period. Some years later, it can be extended to sixty-two days. Some of my patients are on a seventy-two-day treatment. Yet in the light of present knowledge, it appears that stretching the treatment beyond sixty-two days lessens the beneficial effects of menstruation. Excessively long cycles allow the uterine lining to build up and thicken. Some authorities believe that the thickened, congested tissues may offer a foothold to possible cancers. More frequent cleansing of the womb through menstrual flow is advisable as a cancer-preventive. Moreover, the progestins associated with menstrual activity also appear to have a cancer-preventive effect on the tissues of the breast. To lengthen the induced menstrual cycle by a treatment extending beyond sixty-two days is to lose these salutary effects.

The possibility of spacing the menstrual periods almost at will is indeed a great convenience. The sixty-two-day induced cycle works out to only about five menstruations yearly. This appears to be an optimum for older women. (Younger, pre-menopausal women under hormone therapy naturally should follow the normal twenty-eight-day cycle.) But for older women, five menstruations per year is usually all that is needed to relieve menopausal and post-menopausal symptoms, to restore a general sense of well-being, and to brighten the mental outlook and attitude.

Women who have previously experienced painful menstruation need have no fear about the recurrence of discomfort. Once ovulation has ceased, menstrual pain is most unlikely. And so a post-menopausal woman is made to menstruate again with an almost guaranteed absence of any pain whatever.

CASE 6. You are long past menopause and in serious mental and physical difficulties. To name just a few aspects of the total syndrome: deep untractable depression bordering on melancholia, crippling osteoporosis (brittleness of the bones), cholesterol content of the blood so high as to produce imminent danger of strokes or heart attack. You already have experienced a slight cerebral accident or cardiac episode. In such an extreme condition, your vaginal smear is likely to show no estrogen at all. Your Femininity Index is zero.

The treatment in this case might be termed a "crash program" to alleviate an urgent critical situation. The details of the treatment are somewhat involved, and since they may vary according to the individual patient's requirements, no specific routine can be outlined here. If your doctor is not fully acquainted with this technique, he can obtain pertinent information from sources listed in the Medical Appendix to this book.

This type of "crash program" is also indicated in certain special situations when an older woman in poor physical condition is planning to marry a healthy, vigorous man. If such a woman has not enjoyed the benefit of previous estrogen therapy, her vagina may be partially atrophied, pain-sensitive, and nondistensible. She will be inadequate to meet the sexual demands of marriage. Until recently, no doctor could have helped her. Yet today's intensive estrogen therapy may enable her to fulfill all her wifely functions.

The six typical cases postulated above illustrate the principles of therapy for women in different age groups. Thousands of *actual* cases attest to the efficacy of these methods. From the great number of women whose physical and psychic femininity has been successfully retained or restored, let me report but two. I deliberately chose two unusual situations because they seemed virtually hopeless at the outset.

R.M. was a cultured Englishwoman of seventy-two, quite rich, who became attached to a healthy man of fifty-nine while visiting the United States. The two were planning to marry. Except for mild hypertension, she enjoyed basically good health. On her first visit to my office she seemed in a state of considerable disquiet. The marriage was to take place in three weeks, but Mrs. M. had agonizing doubts that it could be physically consumated. A physical examination revealed that her fears were by no means groundless. Her former husband had been killed in World War II some ten years before and she had had no sexual encounters since. A thin, partially atrophied vagina seemed to forestall all hope of a physical union.

I placed Mrs. M. on a massive regimen of estrogen: a daily dose of one-tenth milligram of ethinyl estradiol (an extremely potent semi-natural estrogen), supplemented by hypodermic injections of estradiol benzoate every three or four days. In addition, I prescribed estrogen in the form of vaginal suppositories and frequent external applications of an estrogen cream. An examination three weeks later showed an almost miraculous rejuvenation of her sexual organs. The pathologically dry, unyielding vagina had changed into a perfectly normal, supple, and resilient duct. Her breasts had become firm and sensitive to touch. Her general muscle tone had improved remarkably, and her energy and mental disposition had taken such an upswing that she hardly seemed the same person I had seen at the first consulation.

The marriage took place and—from a physical point of view—it proved successful. Ultimately she and her husband did not get along too well because of the great cultural difference in their backgrounds. But neither of them felt that their marriage was a failure. For both of them it proved an acceptable refuge from a deep loneliness that had threatened to engulf their later years. In a recent letter she explained to me that it was their initial physical contact—so deeply gratifying after years of loneliness—that had set up between them a mutual bond strong enough to withstand the strain of their many differences.

Another case illustrating remarkable recovery from a severe situation is that of Mrs. T. R., aged fifty-three. Both her ovaries had been removed in 1938 because of cysts. As a result, she had not menstruated for twenty-two years when I accepted her as a patient in 1960.

Due to the stoppage of her natural feminine functions at a relatively early age, and the accompanying estrogen deficiency, she had developed hypertension, constant depression, extreme muscle weakness, and advanced osteoporosis of the spine with persistent backaches. These aches were so severe that they literally made her life unendurable. She frequently contemplated suicide through an overdose of barbiturates, which her doctor had prescribed to help her sleep during prolonged periods of acute pain.

When she was referred to me by the orthopedic surgeon who had ineffectually treated her backaches up to then, I immediately put her on a crash program of estrogen and progestin. Despite the fact that she had been—physiologically speaking—castrated for twenty-two years, she responded at the end of the third cycle of massive hypodermic estrogen medication and has been menstruating regularly ever since on double the usual maintenance dose of estrogen and progestin (two and a half milligrams of conjugated estrogens and twenty milligrams of medroxyprogesterone acetate). Her backache disappeared permanently after three weeks of therapy. A year later I was able to demonstrate by X-ray that her formerly porous bones had re-calcified—an exceptional finding. Thanks to the regained strength of her bones, she was able to return to full-time work as a secretary. She still gets depressed occasionally, but no more so than is consistent with her naturally pensive temperament. She never sinks into those glum, suicidal moods characteristic of her former condition. In 1964, four years after the onset of therapy, her blood pressure had dropped a reassuring thirty points to an altogether normal reading of 128/85.

Thousands of additional cases could be cited to buttress arguments in favor of estrogen therapy. Most of them would lack the dramatic extremes of the two instances I have singled out. The bulk of my medical records tell of women in comparatively normal life situations. The files include women of all ages, from their late teens to their eighties, widely differing in physique, personality, and sexual habits. The one thing they have in common is the desire to safeguard their natural femininity and, concomitantly, their total physical and psychological health.

In summary, then, the evidence of medical records now available established the following conclusions:

1. In the vast majority of cases, the distressing bodily changes following menopause are reversible through estrogen treatment. Virtually all the symptoms described in previous chapters can be rectified under consistent estrogen therapy. The skin becomes supple again, the muscles regain their tone and strength, the breasts are restored to almost their former firmness and contours, the genitals again become supple and distensible, skin cracks and genital inflammations heal. Bones that have become brittle regain most of their former strength.

Only one common post-menopausal change is not usually reversible. Once a spinal hump (dowager's hump) has developed, estrogen alone cannot straighten the curved back. Great improvement, however, can be gained when estrogen therapy is combined with proper postural exercises.

As for the psychological complications that usually follow the menopause, estrogen therapy has brightened the outlook of most patients and restored their previous levels of vitality and interest in life. It has also helped them in their personal adjustments both to members of their families and in job situations. To be a woman once more has saved many a post-menopausal patient from neuroses, alcoholism, and other personality disorders.

It should be emphasized that the restoration of normal bodily functions does not prolong fertility beyond its natural span. The fact that menstruation continues does not mean that the woman is fertile. Menstruation continues because the normal chemical cycle of estrogen and a progestin is supplied through medication. But these substances do not replace the egg itself. Once each ovary has delivered its predestined number of eggs, fertility cannot be restored. The use of estrogen-progestin therapy will not prolong fertility by a single day.

2. The medical record proves further the value of preventive treatment. If estrogen therapy is started *before* the onset of menopause, no menopausal symptoms ever develop. The woman simply con-

tinues her normal feminine life without any change at all, except the natural cessation of fertility.

3. Estrogens have proved successful in correcting genital deficiencies and their psycho-sexual consequences at any age—even in young women.

4. The optimum estrogen dosage for any individual woman is readily determined and maintained by a differential cell count in a smear taken from the upper third of the vaginal passage, noting the proportion of superficial cells relative to the number of intermediate and parabasal cells. This count, expressed as a percentage, is a clinically accurate measure of the estrogen level within the system and may be regarded, physiologically speaking, as an index of femininity.

The count is extremely reliable, except in special cases where a local infection exists or where cortisone or other steroids are being administered as a treatment for other conditions.

Thanks to the simple and completely painless way of performing this test, every woman can be assured that the estrogen dosage prescribed is suited to her individual requirements. A twice-a-year check serves to maintain the estrogen level—and hence the Femininity Index—at the optimum.

Before you embark on the great adventure of preserving or regaining your full femininity, your doctor should make you aware of certain medical factors which are quite common in the course of estrogen therapy but which might worry you unless you were previously alerted to them.

Occasionally the therapeutic routine causes slight bleeding between the regular periods. This also happens sometimes to women taking contraceptive pills.

Possibly your first impulse after noticing the slight bleeding is to omit or cut down your estrogen dosage. But this is precisely the wrong thing to do and will increase the amount of bleeding. On the contrary, the bleeding indicates that the estrogen level at that particular time is not quite sufficient to prevent the breakdown of the uterine lining. As your doctor will tell you, you should increase the estrogen intake at such times so that a proper hormonal balance is attained and the untimely bleeding stops. Usually your doctor will double your regular dose during the time of unexpected bleeding. After your next menstruation, you may go back to your normal dose unless the bleeding occurs again.

Some doctors refine the routine by prescribing gradually increasing amounts of estrogen during each cycle. This always prevents bleeding between regular periods.

If the untimely bleeding occurs during the time span when you are taking both estrogen and progestin tablets, it will be most quickly stopped by doubling the dose of progestin. This countermeasure is even more effective than doubling the dose of estrogen.

Some women express concern that menstrual bleeding after menopause induced by estrogen therapy may hide the presence of uterine cancer. Such fears appear groundless when you consider the following:

The regular menstrual flow cleanses the uterus, eliminating congested tissues that are a possible breeding ground of cancers. In effect, the continuation of the menstrual cycle beyond menopause makes it difficult if not impossible for an endometrial cancer (cancer of the uterine lining) to take hold and continue to grow.

The therapy itself provides a form of cancer test. For instance, if bleeding between periods can be stopped by increased or doubled doses of estrogen or progestin, as described above, a malignancy is highly improbable. If the between-period bleeding cannot be stopped in this way, it serves as a danger signal.

But there is little chance of such danger. Women who are amply supplied with estrogen and progestin and who menstruate regularly almost never develop cancer of the uterine lining. The cause of bleeding may be a relatively harmless polyp—a common non-malignant type of growth. In any case, consult your doctor immediately if between-period bleeding does not stop after the taking of additional estrogen or progestin. Very likely, he will suggest a curettage of the uterus to dispel any uncertainty.

Before ending this chapter on the restoration of womanhood through estrogen therapy, a special situation must be considered. What about women who have undergone hysterectomy?

After explaining to a new patient the principle of estrogen therapy, I occasionally hear her despairing outcry: "But doctor, I no longer have a uterus!"

I then assure her that her previous hysterectomy in no way prevents her from enjoying the boon of restored femininity. Whether or not your womb has been removed has no direct bearing on the general medical and psychological benefits to be derived from estrogen.

During numberless medical interviews with women, I have encountered much confusion and misinformation regarding the practice of hysterectomy and ovariectomy. It may therefore be advisable to review these procedures briefly in relation to estrogen therapy.

The uterus may be removed either entirely or in part. In case of a so-called sub-total or supra-cervical abdominal hysterectomy, the cervix—the lower part of the uterus which opens into the vagina—is left in place. Sometimes one ovary and Fallopian tube are removed along with the uterus; sometimes both tubes and ovaries are excised. There are other variants of this basic type of surgery, but they are not relevant to our discussion.

The sole function of the uterus is to form the cradle in which the child ripens for birth. Other than for reproduction, the womb serves no purpose. Once a woman has resolved not to have any more children, or if she is past child-bearing age, the uterus becomes totally useless to her. At best, it is nothing but a nuisance; at worst, an imminent danger.

The non-functional uterus is annoying because the monthly breakdown of the uterine lining causes the various discomforts of menstruation; its danger lies in its being a possible breeding ground for cancer. This is the reason why many women have their wombs removed.

The medical profession is decidedly hesitant about recommending hysterectomy as a general preventive routine. However, it may be that in the future such prophylactic surgery will become acceptable.

The point to remember in the light of our present discussion is that—contrary to popular notions—the center of a woman's femininity is not in her womb but in her ovaries. The womb produces no hormones. As far as the female endocrinology is concerned, it is completely inert. It is the ovaries that produce those vital hormonal substances—estrogen and progesterone— that make a woman feminine.

A woman who has had her uterus removed but retains her ovaries thus appears fortunate indeed. Assuming that her ovaries function normally, she remains fully feminine and enjoys complete freedom from fear of uterine cancer, unwanted pregnancy, and is permanently rid of menstrual annoyances. She is truly an emancipated woman.

Four simple rules can be set down concerning the presence or absence of a uterus in regard to estrogen therapy:

1. If a vaginal smear shows that your Femininity Index is below par and that you are deficient in estro-

gen, the lacking estrogen must be supplied through therapy—regardless of whether you have a uterus or not, and regardless of whether you have one ovary, two ovaries, or none.

2. If you menstruate regularly, this alone is a sign that you have a sufficient supply of progesterone. No specific test is needed. If you menstruate irregularly or not at all, you must replace the lacking progesterone by taking progestin tablets. The woman whose uterus has been removed must also replace the lacking progesterone in this way, regardless of whether she has one ovary, two ovaries, or none.

3. If you still have a uterus, estrogen therapy will induce cyclic bleeding beyond the time when it otherwise would have ceased. This is an inconvenience you must accept in return for the many benefits of the therapy.

4. If your uterus has been removed, estrogen therapy will provide all its benefits without the annoyance of menstrual bleeding. You are a lucky woman indeed.

7

Plain Talk About Sex

By THE TIME my reputation as a specialist in the subtler aspects of gynecology enabled me to practice on Park Avenue, I had acquired the habit of making a special mark on some of the file folders containing my patients' medical records. The mark was a little three-pointed star. It's a pity this emblem hasn't yet become a standard form of medical notation. To me the little star denoted an important clinical fact: it meant the woman was deeply in love with her husband.

Whether a woman is, or has been, in love, I consider essential medical information. My own practice has convinced me that lack of love in a woman's life can be as devastating to her body as any microbe.

The clinical test I developed for ascertaining my patient's state of heart is very simple. I just asked. Of course, I always chose a moment when the question would catch her unawares. And then I watched for her reaction.

A straight "Yes" doesn't mean a thing. But one can usually tell from facial expression or certain other telltale signs whether she belongs to those happy twenty percent (or thereabouts) who really love their husbands. They are my favorite patients. In all menopausal complaints, their prognosis under estrogen treatment is excellent, because, in all matters pertaining to sex, love is the best medicine.

Some women who do not love their husbands will say so with a brutal forthrightness. Their frankness is, perhaps, admirable; but a bland "No" of this kind is literally so chilling that it makes me want to turn off the air conditioner in the middle of summer.

Yet the majority of women when asked, "Do you love your husband?" cannot give a straight answer.

"I respect him very much."

"He is a very good man."

"He is very kind to me."

That's one set of common responses. They don't qualify for the three-pronged star, but the prognosis is still good. But the answers may run like this:

"He's very busy—I don't see him very much."

"He is so tired—even falls asleep at the television set."

"He is not well—wish he would take off some weight and take better care of himself."

Usually these remarks are uttered without any emotion. I know then that something besides estrogen is needed to restore this woman to a fully feminine role. Some plain talk about sex, I found, is a good prescription even for women of menopausal age.

Relations between husband and wife are too vast a

topic to be treated peripherally in any book. And this book, after all, is concerned mainly with the elimination of menopause rather than marital adjustment. The two, however, are inevitably related. And though I cannot, within the scope of this book, develop a complete theory of marital adjustment (especially since I firmly believe that this is not primarily a medical matter but one of mind and spirit), I should like to offer a few observations that might not be readily obtained from the usual sources.

The most common topic of clinical sex talk with mature women is frigidity. Most women think they are frigid if they do not reach a climax during intercourse. They do themselves an injustice. Sexual satisfaction for women takes a far greater range and variety of forms than for men. Outright orgasm is only one of these forms. Many women derive a high degree of satisfaction from lovemaking without orgasm. They may not usually achieve the same degree of relaxation from their lovemaking as do women capable of complete orgasm, yet to describe failure to attain orgasm as frigidity is an arbitrary overstatement.

Most women who do not achieve orgasm do not even mention this fact among their complaints. It has to be elicited by sympathetic questioning. They seldom seem very concerned about it, probably because what they have never experienced, they do not miss. Orgasm plays an exaggerated role as a symbol of fulfillment in contemporary literature, just as making a million dollars used to be a symbol of fulfillment in the old Horatio Alger type of novels. In clinical medicine, however, female orgasm just isn't that important.

Still, though a million dollars isn't necessary, it's nice to have. And so it is with orgasm. In this respect, too, estrogen proves helpful. If, for instance, you have never experienced orgasm and your Femininity Index reveals that you are below par in terms of female sexuality—, say, with sixty percent superficial cells or less—your doctor might prescribe enough estrogen to bring your Index up to the normal eighty percent or more. There's a good chance that the extra estrogen will, so to speak, push you over the brink in your lovemaking.

But if your husband is clumsy or inconsiderate, all the hormones in the world won't help you make up for his faults. So don't blame yourself, but help your husband do a better job. You can do this in various ways. Sex handbooks can be of some help, but they can also be a source of additional frustration. Too often, such books describe the joys of love in prose far too purple for any attainable reality. They incite men to strive for and women to expect the impossible. No happiness can come of that.

Like any book attempting to teach a physical skill, books on how to make love have a built-in drawback. For instance, a man may read a dozen books on how to play golf. But he'll still need some practice out on the course. Sex, for a man, is a physical skill that takes time to develop. Mishaps are bound to occur, along with some of the better things. A wife, especially a

new one, is apt to make a man nervous. She is an unknown destiny on which he has gambled a good part
of his life. New situations will arise, embarrassments
and crises occur, constant adjustments must be made,
and no two people in the world can remain unchanged
by the experience of a maturing marriage. To both
partners, marriage is a surpassing adventure. But it is
the man who must accept most of the sexual challenge.
He is the one who must learn to conduct the active
part of intercourse in a delicate process of trial and
error. The woman's more passive part carries no similar responsibility. Considering the complexity of a
man's sexual task, wives, in all stages of life, should be
extremely careful never to damage their husband's
confidence, never to criticize directly his sexual errors.
Encouragement is needed, and, above all, a sense of
humor. These are the roads that lead to sexual compatibility—and such compatibility is the best antidote
for divorce. Ask any lawyer.

Before discussing differences between male and
female sexual attitudes, it may be advisable to return
once more to that female bugaboo of frigidity. During
the many years in which I practiced what might be
called psychosomatic gynecology, I was never able to
approach the problem of frigidity in terms of stereo-
typed medical procedure. I felt that it must be dealt
with in the broadest term of human experience.

To be sure, any patient who came to me complaining of serious frigidity was given a thorough examination to determine the status of her general health, her

hormonal condition—not merely with regard to estrogen but also in respect to thyroid, pituitary, and adrenal secretions. After these physical factors are ascertained, one must probe for possible mental blocks against normal sexual functioning.

Quite often a kind of sexual paralysis results in a woman who has had a traumatic sex experience in childhood or who had uncommonly strong emotional attachments to her parents. Homosexual tendencies, conscious or otherwise, must be explored. A religious background that pictures sex as sinful often creates a severe block. Even without this kind of indoctrination, the remnants of Puritan philosophy instill a notion that sex is dirty, filthy, and low. Certainly a woman exposed to such influences will have difficulty in her sexual adjustment.

But all these cultural and pseudo-religious handicaps can be overcome by that one overriding three-pronged star factor I marked on my patient's record. I believe that no physically healthy woman who is truly in love is frigid. The apparently frigid woman is simply one who has not fallen in love. In her mind, she carries an image of some ideal man different from her husband. She can settle for nothing less. And she has too much of a fierce, elemental, womanly pride to employ that ageless strategem of prostitutes: to pretend to herself that the man she is with is the man she really wants. Her emotional responses are "all or none."

I have questioned many seemingly-frigid women about that unknown man in the back of their minds who keeps them from enjoying the men they know. I have been amazed to find that he seems to be very much the same man for most such women. He is tall, commanding in posture, he has light, curly hair (eighty to ninety percent of the women I questioned are agreed on this), bright blue eyes, is neither thin nor stout, has perfect teeth and lots of money. Few women seem to care whether he is particularly handsome or not, but on one set of characteristics they all insist: he must be kind, gentle, chivalrous, and brave.

Granted, that's not a bad bet for any girl. But hankering for some fairy-tale knight that has been slipped into her subconscious by a thousand years of legend is a poor reason for closing the door on her available options. It almost seems that such women, by remaining frigid to their real-life husbands, subconsciously try to remain virginal for their ideal mate. A few lucky ones eventually realize that virginity really has nothing to do with the case—either in the real world or the world of their imagination.

One patient of mine made the best of both these worlds.

"I'm marrying a man for his money," she announced one day. Seeing my frown, she added: "What's so wrong about that? I'll be a good wife; he won't regret it. I can wait no longer for the right man to come along. I'm thirty-three. But if he should happen to appear some day, no husband and not all the money in the world would keep me from him."

Her marriage, while lacking that rare quality of rapturous bliss, was a good and happy one, for she was an honest woman. She knew she struck a bargain and was generous with herself and to herself. That's not love, but maybe it's the next best thing.

Contrary to popular belief, the challenge of mutual sexual adjustment is not confined to newlyweds. It continues as long as marriage itself, changing its aspects at various stages of life. With the lengthening of a woman's span of sexual competence by means of estrogen therapy, the need for satisfactory sex techniques and customs continues into later life. To arrive at such techniques, and to modify them according to one's stage in life, it is necessary to understand the essential difference between male and female sexuality.

The first requirement for any happy sex relationship is to regard the subject in the light of healthful decency, to treat sex as a normal aspect of life, and to recognize the sexual element as one of the fundamental components of human nature—in fact, of almost all living things. Considered in this light, sex never needs apology. No shame is connected with it. This applies equally to men and women.

The divergence between men and women is in the manifestations of the sexual impulse. A healthy man's sex is always near the surface of his consciousness. He is sexually aware, even aroused, at the slightest provocation. For him, sex never simmers down to just another biological function. Sex serves him as a kind of mental radar that helps him perceive and interpret the world around him.

For most women, sex is not so external, so outgoing, or so constantly in their awareness. A young bride-to-be who had come to me for a pre-marital examination expressed the more distant attitude toward sex typical of many women. This virginal girl, genuinely looking forward to marriage, was yet able to remark coolly during the examination: "I don't see why people make such a fuss about sex—you'd think it had just been invented."

To a woman, I reflected, sex is always an age-old, inward thing. Even an inexperienced girl has a quiet, resigned acceptance of it that prepares her for the demanding mission of motherhood.

An individual woman's response to sex varies largely according to her childhood conditioning, parental attitudes, early sex shocks, etc. But to women, generally, sex is just another biological function, like eating and sleeping. When regularly exercised, it relieves tension and fills her with a sense of satisfaction. But, except when she is actually engaged in a sexual situation, it does not obtrude itself on her mind.

For a man, by contrast, sex has indeed "just been invented." For him it is always a new discovery, from moment to moment. "Sex is to a man what gnats are in summer," one of my patients once complained. "It bugs them all the time."

The man's quicker, more acute sexual response is conditioned by both his mind and his body. To adjust this response to the slower time factors in the female is for him a task of enormous difficulty. Curiously, the more physical fascination a woman holds for a man, the more difficult it becomes for him to give her the pleasure she deserves and he wants to give. His effort to alter his own bodily reactions in order to give pleasure to his wife deserves all the help a woman can give.

Such help can take many forms. The most effective way to prevent premature ejaculation, I believe, is to retain an aura of romance for one's conjugal exercises. A bored husband, for whom the sex act has become merely a domestic routine—like mowing the lawn—will hardly be inspired toward any kind of sexual exertion to increase his wife's pleasure. A pleasant atmosphere, relaxation, cleanliness, and perhaps a drop of perfume can do a lot to restore an atmosphere of courtship and festivity even after many years of marriage. Under such conditions, fewer husbands would be indifferent or gross.

The manner in which a woman dresses at home and elsewhere also has a considerable effect on her husband's attitude toward her. Most women would do well to remember that only an exceptionally graceful seventeen-year-old girl gains advantage from a bikini. Nudity, in most cases, repels rather than attracts. This simple truth is recognized in all the more elegant bordellos of the Latin world, where one finds exquisite girls exquisitely dressed. Most wives could draw a lesson. Clothes do not have to be elaborate or expensive.

But they should be appealing and tasteful at all times.

Perhaps a doctor should stick to prescribing medicine instead of prescribing fashion. Yet I cannot in good conscience ignore the matter of dress. Trivial as it may seem, it is part of the total aspect of sexuality and marital adjustment. In particular, the recent trend toward stretch pants for casual wear seems, to me at least, diabolically designed to stamp out mature sex. If the average woman could contemplate the vista she presents from astern, she would no longer wonder at her husband's lack of ardor. Clothes are part of a woman's charm, and they should be chosen with precisely that object in mind. Too many of today's fashions strike me as distinctly anti-sexual, because, by an excess of revelation, they destroy the charm and the sense of mystery that stimulate men. If a woman lacks the sense or taste to dress attractively, I believe that her husband should insist on suitable mode of dress for her. This may contribute considerably toward marital harmony.

In dress, as in other matters, the guiding principle should be to retain a woman's femininity despite the current trend toward masculinization. If a wife goes too far in assuming a masculine role or appearance, can she blame her heterosexual husband for loss of libido or even outright impotence? She makes her husband feel that he's sleeping with another man.

The perfection of physical love is, of course, a gradual process, often taking many years. I have known of couples who, after ten years of happy married life, have developed techniques of intercourse in which the man's climax is withheld for as long as an hour, during which the wife experiences several orgasms of varying intensity.

These ultimate heights of sexual joy are, surprisingly, not usually achieved in youth. Rather, they seem to be the prerogative of well-adjusted couples in the middle years, usually around the onset of menopause. In addition to maturity of mind, one of the contributing factors toward these achievements is that the woman is freed from possible fears of pregnancy and any need for contraceptive devices. (In the years before the development of oral chemical contraceptives (see Chapter 9), the insertion of mechanical contraceptives has often had a depressant effect on a woman's sexual responsiveness.)

The most important single factor, however, toward the achievement of sexual satisfaction is an atmosphere of mutual appreciation between the partners, an absence of criticism or recrimination. In such an atmosphere, female orgasm of some degree will nearly always be achieved eventually, often quite unexpectedly.

This atmosphere of mutual appreciation depends, to a large degree, on the ability to express affection. Men and women also differ significantly in this respect. Affection is vital to a woman; in fact, in some instances it can even replace the need for sex. Deprive a wife of affection, and she is truly starved.

Man, by contrast, is not naturally affectionate. This is an unfortunate defect—partly induced by a culture which has always held male participation in war to be one of man's most noble purposes. Man's lack of affectionateness naturally presents serious problems to women. To make matters worse, men tend to become even less affectionate as the years pass. The exact opposite occurs with women, whose need to express affection usually grows with advancing age. Here, incidentally, we have one of the best indicators of the general marital climate. As long as the wife bestows affection on her husband, the marriage is basically healthy. If she withholds affection for a considerable span of time, it signals serious trouble.

When I lecture on the new possibilities of prolonging a woman's femininity into later life, a question is always posed by the audience: "But what about the men?" If women's sexuality is indefinitely prolonged, they ask, can the men keep up with them?

As I have pointed out before, men retain their sexuality until quite late in life. In contrast to untreated women, there is no sudden decline in middle life. At his best, the aging male, if he is in good basic health and takes good care of himself, may have lost some of his hair, but he still carries himself erect. There is nothing apathetic about him. His eyes can flash fire, show scorn or hate, or delight at beauty. His face may be lined, but it is not wrinkled. If such a man has enough interests in life to sustain his spirit, his body will not let him down. He may still swim, fish, golf, or hike, and his mind still welcomes new knowledge and ideas.

But far too many men are more like the husband described by one of my patients: "He comes home so tired. He doesn't want to talk. He's not even interested in the children. He reads the paper at dinner time, then goes to the TV set, takes off his shoes, and falls asleep."

I am sure many women will recognize the pattern. Is this the gracefully aging male—erect, sprightly, and capable?

Clearly there is something wrong here. But it's not likely to be a lack of hormones in a man. More probably, it's a lack of interest. The man is simply bored. The fault may be a dull mind, a dull job, or a dull wife. Whatever it is, it is unendurable and deadly. At the same time, it is a challenge. Both husband and wife must face it and overcome it if their lives are to have meaning and beauty.

Psychiatric counseling may be necessary in a case like this to get to the roots of a husband's passivity. Simple worry may often reduce an otherwise lively man to such a condition. He may worry about being fired, about being in debt, about office politics, about his investments or the tax bill. These worries must be resolved or else they will prevent him from attaining the relaxation and the sense of well-being necessary for a satisfactory marital and sexual relationship. The sex act involves highly complex coordination of nervous and chemical processes within the body. A man exhausted by pressure, conflict, and worry cannot be a good husband. Where circumstances permit it, my prescription for such a couple is a two-month Mediterranean cruise.

Not even the healthiest man, however, retains his sexual functions indefinitely. By the time he reaches sixty-five, he may have experienced a gradual decline of his sexual abilities and he may require medical assistance if he wishes to continue a fully sexed life. In principle, the same therapy applies to him as to women. The gradually diminishing sex hormones must be supplied through medication. Excellent male steroids are now available by injection, implantation of pellets, or as tablets for this form of therapy. The continuing or restoration of male sexuality, however, are separate topics that fall outside the scope of this book.

In conclusion I should like, however, to touch upon a common male anxiety that often interferes with proper sexual performance. Men often worry about the (presumably inadequate) size of their penis. This type of worry is reinforced by a peculiar folklore that has nothing whatever to do with physiological reality. The vagina, being highly elastic, accommodates itself readily to almost any penis dimensions, and a woman's sensations during intercourse are evidently far less affected by penis size than is commonly assumed. Men might take comfort from the fact that in all my years as a gynecologist, I never once encountered a woman who complained about the size of her husband's penis.

8

A Matter of Education Versus Prejudice

I AM CERTAIN this book will be attacked in some quarters, not perhaps on medical grounds, but because of my polemic attitude. A doctor is not supposed to plead and argue—merely to state facts.

Facts, indeed, ought to suffice; and I trust that I have presented conclusive evidence in favor of estrogen therapy.

But I have learned that, unfortunately, in my field of research—sex and hormones—myth and prejudice often outweigh reason, and evidence is obscured by prejudice. The purely rational presentation of clinical fact must therefore be supplemented by an educational effort to rout entrenched misconceptions.

"You're doing the devil's work!" a minister once snapped at me during a lecture. To prolong normal married life and conjugal happiness was to him a sin. It didn't matter to him that the primary purpose of estrogen therapy is to assure a woman's general health.

He only saw S-E-X, which he evidently regarded as the motto inscribed upon the Gates of Hell.

"But is not marriage a sacrament?" I asked. "Have you not yourself solemnized marriage as a minister? My branch of medicine merely helps the church in maintaining health and harmony in marriage." The man of God merely snorted and turned on his heels.

Most clerics, however, have been sympathetic to my work. Knowing through their counseling work the depth of domestic misery often brought on by un-treated menopause—ministers, priests, and rabbis are often more receptive to the idea of hormone therapy than the more traditional-minded members of my own profession.

The most enlightened response I have ever encoun-tered from clerical quarters came from the Mother Su-perior of a convent. She had been referred to me through St. Mary's Hospital in Brooklyn, where I have been a staff member since 1938, because she wanted to discuss a regular program of estrogen ther-apy for her older nuns, simply as a preventive health measure.

Such informed intelligence is rare. Far too many persons, even today, still carry traces of ancient super-stitions and taboos concerning women that have been rooted in the human mind for thousands of years.

Most of these myths stem from the fact that the nature of the menstrual flow was not understood until quite recently. The ancient Greeks and Romans re-garded menstruation as a sign of evil and uncleanli-ness, a "curse" laid upon women. They believed that crops would wither if touched by a menstruating woman. Even an otherwise remarkable naturalist, Pliny the Elder, wrote of menstruation in a "scientific" treatise in the first century of the Christian era: "On approach of a woman in that state, new wine turns sour, seeds touched by her become sterile, grass withers away, garden plants are parched up, and the fruit will fall from the tree beneath which she sits."

Through the ages, the same theme reverberates. A poet of medieval England sang:

> Oh! Menstruating woman, thou'rt a fiend
> From whom all nature must be screened!

As late as 1878—less than a hundred years ago—the scientific *British Medical Journal* declared blandly: "It is an undoubted fact that meat spoils when touched by menstruating women." Even in this century, sugar refineries in France forbade menstruating women workers to enter the plant for fear that their presence would turn the sugar black. To this day, many French provincial women will not try to mix sauce or mayonnaise during their menstrual periods, themselves convinced that their "curse" would spoil their cooking.

The Jews even put their fear of menstruation into religious laws. Women of extreme orthodox persuasion must take ritual baths after each menstrual period, and any person touched by a woman before this bath is defiled.

The religious concern lavished upon women—at least in the past—was anything but sympathetic. Traditionally, Judeo-Christian theologians viewed woman as an "unclean vessel." As a physician, I have never been able to comprehend how pious men could be so lacking in appreciation of God's marvelous design and workmanship in making the human body.

While these beliefs about women are gradually fading in the light of modern medical knowledge about the female sex cycle, an aura of old-wives' tales still clings to what is coyly called "the change of life." The very phrase is typical of the Victorian determination to call a spade anything but a spade. As regards menopause, the old fears and fables are still with us. Only now these fears have a new focus: hormone therapy.

The opposition I have encountered to hormone therapy is, for the most part, so utterly irrational and so blind to evidence that I feel these objections are in essence a new facet of the ancient anti-feminine prejudice. Fear of the devil, to be sure, is no longer invoked in denying women the full possibilities of life. Instead two new bogeys are set up: fear of breast and uterine cancer, and fear of masculinization due to hormone therapy.

Both these topics have been discussed in previous chapters, and I have cited evidence to establish two vital points:

1) Estrogen therapy, far from causing cancer, tends to prevent it.
2) Estrogen, far from causing a change to male characteristics, promotes typically feminine appearance. (It is androgen, the male sex hormone, that is responsible for male appearance.)

In both cases, the truth is exactly the opposite of widespread belief. In view of such tragic misunderstandings, additional explanations may be in order.

I have already cited the report in the *Journal of the American Medical Association* of October 27, 1962, on a group of 304 women treated with estrogen for periods up to twenty-seven years. According to the norm for non-treated women, eighteen cases of breast or uterine cancer would normally be expected in this group. Yet among the estrogen-treated women, not a single case occurred.

The same kinds of results are being now obtained time and again in other studies. Dr. Walter Alvarez, the chief editor of *Geriatrics,* whose popular writings on medical subjects are widely syndicated in newspapers throughout the country, reports: "For the past twenty-five years . . . I have been giving female hormones to hundreds of menopausal women, and so far I haven't seen one develop a cancer that I could blame on the medicine." A recent meeting of the American College of Obstetricians and Gynecologists also went on record saying that the giving of female hormones is not to be feared.

Why then, in the face of such evidence, does so much mistrust still persist toward a form of therapy that spells promise and hope for every woman alive? Part of the answer may be found in a curiously ill-planned and misleading experiment conducted in 1939 by Dr. A. Lacassagne in France. At that time, when hormone and cancer research were both in their infancy, it was found that cancerous growths resulted when certain chemicals were administered to mice. These chemicals included many different substances, among which were a few with estrogenic properties. After these experiments with mice, the generalization was frequently made that any substance with estrogenic properties was "carcinogenic" (cancer-producing).

The accusation that estrogen produces cancer in humans was based on this evidence alone. The publicity for this conclusion was world-wide, and has resounded to the present day.

Little effort has been made, for some unknown reason, to present more than these bare facts. It is time to correct this omission.

A special strain of mouse, which had been inbred for hundreds of generations, was used in these experiments. These mice had a high incidence of spontaneous cancer. Even if *no* chemicals whatever had been administered to them—more than fifty percent of them would have developed cancer. What therefore is proven if, after the injection of an estrogenic chemical, eighty or ninety percent of these abnormally sensitive mice developed cancers? Cancer would undoubtedly have been produced by injections of aspirin, or some other normally harmless medicine. Yet estrogens has been regarded with suspicion on the basis of this laboratory evidence.

And what about dosage?

A mouse weighs about fifty grams and lives two years. The mice in these experiments were given as much as one gram of the estrogenic chemical weekly for six months, or somewhat more than twenty-four grams. Therefore, the amount of the chemical given to the already susceptible mouse was one-half of its body weight administered during one-fourth of its life. It would obviously be impossible to administer a proportionate amount to a human being—even over a twenty-year span.

How naïve, and how inept, researchers were in those days to draw any kind of parallel between a mouse practically drowned in an overdose of estrogens for most of its life and a normal medical situation with highly refined medicines that had not yet even been developed at the time this experiment was carried out. Yet the human mind is so inflexible, so set in its established notions, that the negative image of estrogen created by this experiment has not yet been fully erased.

The conclusion that estrogen causes cancer has never been confirmed in experiments with other animals. No malignant growths were produced when monkeys were assaulted with estrogens (augmented with known carcinogens) for as long as ten years. Other investigators gave massive doses of estrogens to rhesus monkeys for as long as seven years. Some of the monkeys received as much as 1,000,000 rat units a year. Yet there wasn't one case of cancerous change in any organ. Because of the close relationship of monkey to man, these experiments are especially valid in evaluating estrogen in humans.

The world-renowned Dr. Bernard Zondek found that enormous doses of natural estrogens failed to induce growths in rats and in a large number of humans.

Despite the inability of these and many other investigators to produce cancer by means of estrogen in any laboratory animal (except the abnormally susceptible mouse), the mistrust of estrogen continues.

This mistrust is surprising, particularly since there is no convincing proof, in all medical literature, that estrogen has ever induced cancer in a human being.

Another factor to consider is the estrogen concentration in the body relative to the incidence of cancer at various ages. A woman's body, it should be remembered, has possessed estrogen *all her life.* She has received its benefits from even long before birth. From the moment of conception, her destiny has been closely intertwined with it.

There is also the reassuring fact that the greatest amount of estrogen is in a woman's body between the ages of eighteen and twenty-five . . . but breast cancer and cancer of the womb are, during those years, at their lowest incidence.

Actually, the occurrence of cancer of all sites in women increases constantly with age—at the same time that the production of estrogen is steadily declining.

The fanatic believer in the "estrogen menace" refuses to face these facts, since he cannot explain them.

Additional evidence concerning the relation of cancer to estrogen can be obtained from studying the physiologic state of pregnant women.

In the non-pregnant woman, the total estrogen produced during the twenty-eight days of the menstrual cycle is about five milligrams. In the eighth or ninth month of pregnancy, the placenta produces estrogen and pours it into the mother's bloodstream in prodigious amounts.

In the last two months of pregnancy, 3,000 milligrams of estrogenic substances per month enter the circulation—about six hundred times greater than in the absence of pregnancy. This estrogen passes freely into the fetus, and this large supply is now known to be vital to the well-being of the fetus.

You can see from this that malignancy of the breast should be a frequent occurrence in pregnancy, if estrogen were carcinogenic. Yet this is not so.

As I have already pointed out, menstruation in itself appears to have a cancer-preventive effect because any incipient nest of abnormal cells in the womb's lining is mechanically washed away in this cyclic bleeding. Menstruation, far from being a "curse," is therefore closer to a blessing.

Estrogen is sometimes mentioned in relation to cancer of the endometrium (lining of the womb); in regard to this relationship, many people are apparently unaware that ninety-two percent of cases of endometrial cancer occur during or after the menopause—when estrogen levels, already decreased, are declining steadily.

These, then, are facts to keep in mind when you

hear estrogen discussed with suspicion: the inept and illogical mouse experiment that gave rise to the estrogen-cancer myth, and the inverse relationship of estrogen to breast and genital cancer (high estrogen in youth: low cancer incidence . . . low estrogen in age: high cancer incidence).

Keeping a woman rich in her ovarian hormones, estrogen and progesterone, lessens the incidence of malignant lesions, including breast and genital cancer. Certainly, the fear of these cancers need no longer be a factor in the constantly expanding usage of the female sex hormones.

Aside from cancer, the other major fear connected with hormone therapy concerns unwanted side effects. These fears, too, have a historical basis. In the early days of hormone research—from about 1890 to 1920— the field had attracted a number of charlatans and quacks. The existence of hormones had been discovered only a short time before, and specific substances and their effects had yet to be identified. But some doctors were too impatient to await the gradual and orderly advance of medical knowledge. For example, a French doctor named Brown-Séquard claimed to "rejuvenate" males by injecting them with testicular extracts of dogs and monkeys. No matter what other, more rigorous researchers accomplished later, in the public mind, the new science of endocrinology simply meant "monkey glands." The public has yet to realize that, during the past thirty years, endocrinology has developed into one of the most exacting and precise areas of medical research whose benefits are only now beginning to reach large number of patients.

By about 1940, the chemistry of hormones and their various effects was so well understood that unwanted side effects could be eliminated in most medically used hormones. As regards female sex hormones, I have been using conjugated natural estrogens for twenty-five years on thousands of women and have not encountered a single case of allergy. These natural estrogens are so completely metabolized that, under normal conditions, no symptoms of hyperestrinism (over-dosage) ever develop. Cases where estrogen therapy is not recommended are in women with liver disease that might impair their ability to handle the estrogen normally.

As for the masculine appearance of some post-menopausal women, it should be clearly understood that this is caused by lack of estrogen rather than by its presence. The female body normally contains, in addition to the female sex hormones (estrogens and progesterone), small amounts of the male hormone androgen. This is quite normal. Despite the presence of the male hormone, a woman remains feminine as long as she has a *preponderance* of estrogen. It's a matter of proper proportion. Yet with the onset of menopause, the estrogen supply diminishes as the ovaries shrivel. The amount of androgen, however, remains constant. The result is a shift of hormone balance toward the masculine side. That wispy tuft on the upper lip coarsens into a most improper moustache, the woman begins growing fur on her arms and legs and her voice deepens.

"It's because of hormones," the old wives whisper.

They're absolutely right, for once. But it's because *the wrong kind of hormones* have gained domination in the woman's body. The woman needs estrogen to restore the proper female balance.

The point to remember is simply this: estrogen therapy does not cause masculinization in women. On the contrary, it prevents it.

I have explained the relation of hormone therapy to cancer and masculinization to hundreds of patients, and most of them are reassured by the facts I have just cited. Yet a small percentage keep their minds firmly closed.

A case in point is Mrs. S., a faithful patient for over twenty years. Twice yearly she came in for a complete examination, including a Pap Test. She was beset by a pathological fear of cancer and talked of it constantly. Somewhere in her voracious reading on the subject she picked up the old notion that estrogen may produce cancer. Since then she had refused to listen to later findings. She is not unintelligent, but on that subject her mind is closed.

She is sixty years old and has had a Femininity Index of zero (no estrogen) for the past ten years. She is five feet four inches tall, and weighed 134 pounds before menopause. Today she weighs eighty-four pounds and loses weight at the rate of four pounds per year. It is clearly a case of tissue loss caused by negative nitrogen balance due to estrogen deficiency. She, however, blames it on her dentures. She won't agree to hormone treatment aimed at helping her build up her body tissues.

"Hormones are very dangerous," she mutters.

The weight loss obviously cannot continue much longer. In her present weakened condition, even a severe cold could prove fatal. One might diagnose her case as "inadvertent suicide by obstinacy."

I had the cure in my desk drawer, but I could not help her. I had thought of resigning the case. But that would only have upset her and made matters worse. I often wonder how many other women, like her, lose their chance of health and happiness through sheer unreason.

Irrational refusal of hormone therapy also led to tragic results for Mrs. K.B., who entered the hospital at the age of fifty for a routine hysterectomy, because of a fibroid condition in her uterus. Her menopause had occurred five years earlier, and her non-functioning ovaries and tubes were removed along with the uterus. At the time of the operation, she was in good health except for slightly high blood pressure and an extremely high level of cholesterol in her blood. After she was discharged from the hospital, I suggested estrogen therapy to reduce cholesterol and blood pressure. I hoped thereby to forestall a possible stroke or heart attack. I also explained to her the other benefits of estrogen, and she enthusiastically agreed to take the tablets.

For two years afterward she came in for periodic checkups. Estrogen had reduced her blood pressure to normal. Cholesterol registered less than half of the previous reading, and her general health was excellent thanks to the other beneficial effects of estrogen.

Suddenly she stopped seeing me. Members of her family brought disquieting news. Mrs. K.B. had stopped taking estrogen. She had heard it causes cancer. No, she wouldn't listen to anything I had to say. I was a bad doctor for having suggested hormones in the first place.

Two years later her daughter told me that Mrs. K.B. had become emotionally unstable. Alcoholism entered the picture, along with frequent domestic squabbles. The daughter tried to persuade her to resume the estrogen treatments that had served her so well in the past.

"You want to kill me with cancer!" was the shouted reply.

Three years later, the daughter brought news that Mrs. K.B. had died of coronary thrombosis following two previous minor attacks. Evidently her blood pressure and cholesterol level had built up again after she stopped taking estrogen.

Most disheartening to me was the fact that Mrs. K.B. was an intelligent, educated woman, a graduate of Bryn Mawr, who had been at first most receptive to my arguments. She had asked perceptive questions and, I am sure, had understood the medical significance of estrogen treatment. What could have influenced such a woman to succumb to unreasoning fear and to close her mind to evidence? What is it that makes even intelligent women fall victim to myth?

Unreasoning reluctance to accept hormone therapy is, as we have pointed out before, not confined to the uninformed or misinformed public. The medical profession itself, as so often in the past, is slow to make use of new knowledge. The history of medicine is full of unrecognized prophets, missed opportunities, and embarrassed hindsight.

A certain irony lies in the fact that gynecology—the branch of medicine most directly concerned—was by no means the first to recognize, even partially, the merits of estrogen therapy. While most gynecologists maintained an attitude of indifference toward what is undoubtedly the most significant recent advance in their field, it remained for the orthopedic surgeon to exploit the remarkable effects of estrogen. A difficult and obstinate problem facing the orthopedic surgeon is the slow healing of bone fractures in persons of middle age and beyond. Most post-menopausal women make particularly difficult patients in this respect. Their cases are often complicated by osteoporosis, the increasing porosity and brittleness of the bones after menopause. In some cases, this dangerous and painful condition is so advanced as to render bone surgery virtually impossible.

Enlightened orthopedic surgeons had become aware of the restorative effect of estrogen on the bones of middle-aged and older women and adopted the practice of prescribing massive doses of estrogen to their pre- and post-operative patients to speed the healing of fractures.

"I can't understand most of you gynecologists," an orthopedic surgeon chided me once. "You leave it to us surgeons to pump these women full of estrogen to correct their nitrogen unbalance. Frankly, I think some of them are lucky they broke their bones. Otherwise they'd never have got the estrogen."

The remark was made jestingly. But it was a hard rebuke to the medical profession as a whole for its hidebound unwillingness to use new therapeutic methods even when such methods are crucial to the patient's health.

The most unfortunate kind of miseducation is often perpetrated by well-meaning people. The popular author Maxine Davis, for instance, whose widely read guidance books for women are very sensible in most respects, nevertheless repeats many outmoded notions about menopause. In the light of what is clinically known about menopause and of the acute suffering and danger it brings to so many women, what are we to make of the following statement in Miss Davis's *Every Woman's Book of Health:* the menopause "is an event to which a woman can look forward with the happy anticipation of a child waiting for Santa Claus."

What's so good about menopause? Miss Davis tells you: "Only after she reaches her menopause can she count on emotional stability, on remaining for the rest of her adult life on an even keel. No more premen-

strual tension or irritability . . . Every day of the
month she is herself, her best self, and knows that she
can count on her mature abilities."

This statement is exactly the opposite of what we
know to be the truth for at least eighty-five percent of
all women.

Miss Davis goes on: "The menopause is a normal
episode in the life of every woman—normal as morning and evening, normal as summer after spring."

I can only assume that Miss Davis is unaware of the
changes in human life expectancy we have discussed
in the opening chapters, and that menopause, far from
being the evening of life, is much closer to its high
noon. Otherwise she would realize that menopause is
not at all "normal" as a condition of life. She seems
equally unaware, for example, of menopausal effects
on a woman's metabolism and nitrogen balance. How
else could a serious deficiency disease such as menopause seem "normal" to her?

Very likely, like millions of other women, she has
not yet had the opportunity to learn the facts. It is my
own responsibility, however, not to let statements like
hers go unchallenged. That, too, is part of the educational effort which physicians owe to the public.

To end this fusillade at fallacy and falsehood, I
should like to aim a couple of parting potshots at two
minor but very widespread misconceptions. One is
that estrogen therapy is pointless if the patient has had
a hysterectomy. The other is that estrogen therapy is
only for post-menopausal women.

I have already mentioned cases in which estrogen was given with excellent results to women who had had their wombs, their ovaries, or both removed. In fact, whenever the ovaries have been removed—for whatever reason—subsequent estrogen therapy is essential to the woman's health. Since she no longer posesses her chief natural source of estrogen, substitution by externally supplied estrogen becomes necessary. Otherwise she is almost certain to suffer severe symptoms of the kind described in Chapter Five. Whenever a double ovariectomy has been performed, estrogen should be given regardless of the woman's age.

As for hysterectomies (removal of the womb), this operation is becoming increasingly "fashionable" among women who no longer desire to bear children. At times it is advisable as a prophylactic measure against the possibility of uterine cancer. The removal of the womb does not in any way lessen the effectiveness of estrogen therapy. Given sufficient estrogen, a woman whose womb has been removed can still be fully feminine in every respect and enjoy a satisfying sex life. She differs from most other women only in her inability to bear children.

Many women ask me: "What is the proper age to begin estrogen therapy?" My answer invariably is that there is no "proper age." Estrogen may be needed at any age, either before or after menopause. The most practical way to determine this need, and the proper dosage to be given, is through the Femininity Index—the simple test described in Chapter 6.

Quite often, the Femininity Index begins to fall below normal several years before any other signs of approaching menopause are noticed. This frequently happens with women in their middle thirties. If estrogen therapy is begun at that point and continued for life, it provides prophylactic assurance that the woman will never suffer serious menopausal symptoms. I therefore recommend to every woman over thirty that she have her Femininity Index checked once a year. This quick, painless test may prove a turning point in her life, an assurance of continued health and happiness.

I have occasionally encountered underdeveloped women who require estrogen in their twenties, prior to marriage. Such cases, of course, are unusual, though by no means rare. About five percent of women suffer some degree of underdevelopment. Such women are sometimes unable to perform the sexual act simply because their sex organs are not sufficiently distensible to admit the penis.

The most interesting case of this kind I ever encountered was Judith, a tiny, shy, smiling girl of twenty-two, whose manner and appearance suggested a child half her age. She came with her mother and kept clinging to the older woman's hand throughout our first interview. Each time she answered a question, she looked at her mother for confirmation, often asking, "Am I right about that, Mother?"

The reason Judith came to consult me was that she had never menstruated—a fact which caused great concern to her family physician, who had made the referral. Normally I ask women past twenty about their marital status and sex experience, but in Judith's case the question simply seemed absurd. Sex obviously had no meaning to this perennial child.

The circumstances of Judith's life were unusual. As the only child of a well-off couple, she was constantly in the presence of her parents. After dropping out of high school—despite her evident intelligence—she worked as her father's secretary. Her mother worked at the office too. The three were together every day from the time they got up to the time they went to bed. Judith had never had a close girl friend; she had never been out on a date. But, she said, she didn't miss social life.

It was difficult to examine Judith. She was painfully shy, even though her mother had accompanied her into the examination room at her request. I finally was able to ascertain complete sexual underdevelopment— tiny uterus, undeveloped ovaries, undersized breasts. My strong suggestion for a complete endocrinologic survey, carried out in a hospital, was flatly rejected by the patient and her family. As my pleading for such a thorough examination proved of no avail, I reluctantly took recourse to what was the next best possibility. I prescribed large doses of estrogen with balancing amounts of a progestin.

After the first visit I received a phone call from Judith's mother, who volunteered some more information. An intelligent woman, she was fully aware of the fact that Judith had been very much over-protected.

She and her husband had wanted a large family. Consequently they felt great concern about Judith when it became apparent that there would be no more children. Besides, Judith had been a premature baby and had grown up much smaller than other children her age. "She's never so much as had a crush on a boy," she said, "and maybe it's my fault."

I was able to tell Judith's mother quite honestly that whatever the girl's psychological problems may have been, overprotectiveness was certainly not to blame for her hormone deficiency. In fact, I assured her that Judith might have been in a much worse position psychologically if it had not been for her parents' devotion.

"The girl might have become completely withdrawn," I explained, "if you and your husband had not given her some meaningful sphere of functioning and fulfillment within her family." I also suggested that, while hormone treatment would help Judith physically, it would take an exceptionally skilled and experienced psychiatrist to awaken her psychologically to the belated advent of her womanhood. But both Judith and her mother felt that a psychiatrist would constitute an intrusion and a threat to their tightly knit family life and declined my suggestion.

Three months after the beginning of hormone therapy, Judith called me: "It's happened!" she shouted jubilantly. "I'm menstruating!"

Physically, Judith changed visibly from a child into a woman during the following year. She became a little plumper, rounding out her angularities with proper feminine contours. She also seemed happier, and her smile changed from an expression of shyness to an expression of confidence. Her vagina, uterus, and breasts assumed normal proportions, and perhaps the most significant change was that she would allow me to examine her without her mother being present.

Her treatment continued for seven years, during which her social life expanded considerably. She made friends with several other girls, went to movies, to concerts, and occasionally even to a party. But she never dated a young man, and insisted that she wasn't missing anything. Due to the emotional shelteredness of her earlier life, the concept of romance and of falling in love was beyond her, even though she was now physically capable of functioning completely as a woman. If only she had consented to psychotherapy to supplement the hormone treatment, she might have had a full and normal life.

Sexual underdevelopment of this extreme kind may be due to hormonal disturbances more complex than simple estrogen deficiency. I therefore recommend that such patients be examined by an endocrinologist at a hospital offering full diagnostic facilities in this specialty. Unfortunately, relatively few hospitals are equipped to provide a complete endocrinological assay of pituitary, adrenal, ovarian, thyroid, and other secretions. When such facilities are not available, the next best alternative is to take a Femininity Index and then prescribe appropriate amounts of estrogen and a progestin. I have known a number of cases where this simple treatment alone has enabled a sexually under-developed girl to have a normal marriage.

My main concern, however, is the average woman. For her the Femininity Index test, followed, if necessary, by appropriate estrogen and progestin therapy, is the best available means for keeping healthy and normal. The clinical research toward this end is well advanced. What remains to be achieved is the broader application of the results and the mass education of today's woman.

9

Birth Control Pills and Menopause Prevention

FOR ME, THE date is unforgettable. It was the afternoon of February 13, 1963. I was filling out the file card for Mrs. P.G., a new patient who had been referred by her family physician for a routine Pap Test and gynecologic checkup.

"Age?" I asked.

"Fifty-two," the woman said.

After taking down her medical history, I began her physical examination. I was amazed that her body showed almost none of the usual signs of a woman past child-bearing age. Her breasts were supple and firm, her carriage erect; she had good general muscle tone, no dryness of the mucous membranes, and no visible genital atrophy. Above all, her skin was smooth and pliant as a girl's; not even the neck was wrinkled.

I commented on her youthful physique and asked if she had received any hormone treatment after menopause.

"Oh no," she protested. "Our family doctor doesn't

believe in that kind of thing. Besides, I haven't reached menopause yet.

My astonishment must have shown in my face.

"I assure you, Dr. Wilson. I have never yet missed a period." Laughing at my evident surprise, she added: "I'm so regular, astronomers could use me for timing the moon."

This seemed so unusual for a woman of fifty-two that I could hardly wait for the laboratory report on her vaginal cell count. It turned out to be a splendid Femininity Index of ninety percent superficial cells.

Nothing in Mrs. P.G.'s medical or personal history would account for her seemingly unusual youthfulness. The wife of a successful writer, she was a bright, charming woman who led an active social life, was fond of playing golf, and travelled frequently. All her activities were quite normal, and her health record was equally unexceptional.

I was still puzzling about this when one day I received a phone call from her.

"I am sorry to disturb you, Dr. Wilson," her voice came over the wire. "There's one thing I forgot to mention. I thought you might want to know—I've been taking birth control pills for nearly three years. My doctor prescribed them."

At first, this added information seemed merely amusing. A fifty-two-year-old woman still worrying about having babies! On second thought, her concern seemed quite logical. After all, she was still menstruating; consequently she assumed that she was still fertile

although, from a medical point of view, this seemed
highly improbable.

On still further reflection, I finally unraveled the
mystery of the case: it was the birth control pills that
enabled Mrs. P.G. to avoid the menopause.

Soon the logical connection between "the pill" and
the menopause prevention became clear in my mind.
Chemically, there is a close relationship between the
contents of contraceptive pills and the hormones employed in menopause therapy. In some pills, the hormones are identical. One brand of birth control pills
contains a combination of an estrogen (mestranol)
and an *estrogenic progestin* (norethynodrel), both
quite similar to the hormones (estrogen and a progestin) I had been using all along for menopause prevention. It so happened that Mrs. P.G. had been taking
that particular type of pill. Without realizing it, her
doctor had been prescribing monopause therapy—the
very thing of which he disapproved.

This estrogenic birth control pill provides a form of
menopause prevention and treatment in addition to its
contraceptive effect. The chief difference is that in the
usual type of menopause therapy (described in Chapter 6) estrogen and a progestin are given in sequence
during different phases of the menstrual cycle,
whereas the birth control pill contains both estrogen
and a progestin in combination.

It struck me at once that this previously unsuspected property of certain birth control pills (acting as
menopause preventive) may prove to be even more

important than their principal purpose. With approximately six million women in the United States alone now taking oral contraceptives, the possibility of "automatic" menopause prevention through these pills assumes tremendous significance.

Immediately after my encounter with Mrs. P.G., I began a systematic study of contraceptive pills as menopause preventatives. On the basis of my findings, *I can now confidently assert that no woman who uses estrogenic birth control pills (i.e., pills containing norethynodrel) will ever experience menopause if she continues taking "the pill" beyond her childbearing years.*

The principle of "the pill" is to create essentially similar hormonal conditions to those normally preventing ovulation during pregnancy. This hormonal situation makes the pituitary gland act *as if* the woman were really pregnant: no more chemical signals are sent to the ovaries; no more eggs are sent down to the uterus. Hence the woman cannot conceive.

The pill accomplishes this by providing ample amounts of synthetic progestin (an analog of progesterone). Putting both estrogen and progestin in a single package greatly simplifies the routine both for fertility control and for menopause prevention.

It is important to keep in mind that not all fertility control pills now on the market can be used to prevent menopause. Only those which contain a progestin which is inherently estrogenic (e.g., norethynodrel) should be used. Some pills contain progestins which are *not* estrogenic. In fact, they actually are anti-estrogenic, androgenic and masculinizing. These androgenic pills cannot compensate for estrogen deficiency or adequately serve as menopause preventatives.

When I first presented these findings to a medical symposium at Augusta, Georgia, in 1964 under the direction of The Medical College of Georgia, they were received with great interest. But the physiological processes involved were so self-evident that no dissenting opinions were voiced in the ensuing discussion. In fact, one of the world's outstanding authorities in the field of female sex hormones, Dr. John A. Loraine of the University of Edinburgh, Scotland, who had come all the way to Georgia for this symposium, invited me to visit and confer with him and his colleagues at the university on the subject of menopause prevention through birth control pills.

As this is being written, in late 1965, I have just completed an intensive study of eighty-two cases in which menopause was effectively prevented or cured by the use of *estrogenic* birth control pills. The women in my research group ranged from thirty-two to fifty-seven years with an average of 45.8 years. The study represents a total of 132 patient-years and 1591 menstrual cycles. Of twenty-seven patients who took birth control pills specifically to avoid menopause, twenty-six were completely successful. They never developed any menopausal symptoms. The single exception experienced only mild symptoms. The other patients in this group took birth control pills to relieve menopausal symptoms that had already set in. This proved effective in ninety-three percent of these cases.

Along with two co-authors, Dr. Edmund R. Marino and my wife, Thelma A. Wilson, R.N., I have submitted an extensively detailed report of this work to one of our respected and authoritative medical journals, where it awaits publication. To the best of my knowledge, it represents the first scientifically controlled research effort in this new area of medical investigation.

The question naturally arises whether menopause prevention through estrogenic birth control pills is as safe as the older method through separate (sequential) estrogen and progestin tablets as described in Chapter 6.

In the study of eighty-two patients just cited, not a single case of systemic, breast, or genital cancer was observed. Much more significant is the report presented in 1964 by Drs. Gregory Pincus and Celso-Ramon Garcia to the International Union Against Cancer. Their study comprised 5,374 cases of women using contraceptive tablets. None of these women developed cervical cancers after starting the use of the pills—an incidence far below the normal statistical cancer expectancy.

A quite similar study conducted in Puerto Rico by Dr. Adaline P. Satterthwaite and myself on 756 women ranging in age from nineteen to fifty comprised a total of 1517 patient-years and 18,204 menstrual cycles. Statistically 4.2 breast cancers were to be expected in such a group, yet not a single cancer was actually encountered.

The mounting evidence suggests that some types of birth-control pills presently available offer a cancer-preventive effect similar to that already discussed in connection with sequential type (separate estrogen and progestin tablets) of hormone therapy for menopausal symptoms.

Aside from their function in fertility control, estrogenic contraceptive pills thus accomplish three other . . . goals; they: a) keep women estrogen-rich, b) cancer-poor, and c) prevent menopause.

Under no circumstances should birth-control pills be taken without a doctor's approval and supervision. The same warning against self-medication applies here as in the case of separate estrogen and progestin pills.

There is little doubt in the minds of far-seeing doctors, sociologists, and statesmen that fertility control through hormones is among the most significant advances in human health and welfare this century has produced. This marvelous research accomplishment must be credited largely to the Worcester Foundation for Experimental Biology at Shrewsbury, Massachusetts, and in particular to Drs. Gregory Pincus, Celso-Ramon Garcia, and John Rock. Their work constitutes a milestone, not merely in the history of medicine, but in the history of human civilization. Readers interested in fertility research will find the story of the contraceptive pill told with admirable simplicity and accuracy by Albert Q. Maisel in his book *The Hormone Quest*. Mr. Maisel presents the development of "the pill" in the total perspective of hormone research, beginning with the discovery of sex hormones by Arnold Adolph Berthold in Germany more than a hundred years ago. His narrative is replete with human interest and compellingly conveys the sense of adventure that attends almost any kind of vital scientific research. How the various hormones were first recognized and later isolated and synthesized is in itself a fascinating kind of detective story.

Equally intriguing are the economics of hormone therapy. The discoverer of estrogen, Dr. Edward Doisy, had to process the ovaries of more than eighty thousand sows to get just twelve-thousandths of a gram of the precious hormone. Imagine: eighty thousand animals to yield less than a pinhead of pure hormone! At that rate, medical use of the hormone was obviously out of the question. Not even the world's richest woman would have been able to afford a single dose.

Not until a brilliant but eccentric American chemist named Russell Marker found a way of mass-producing certain female sex hormones did modern therapeutic routines become feasible on a large scale.

Marker's career is one of the strangest chapters in the history of modern science. Temperamentally unable to fit himself into any research organization, Marker had walked out of every job he ever held, never bothering about such formalities as a resignation. Even when, by virtue of his unmistakable genius, he was placed at the head of great laboratories, one could never be sure when he left his office that he'd ever come back. And one day he didn't.

Scouting alone in the Mexican wilderness, he was following a hunch. He believed that he could transform the extract of a certain Mexican lily root into progesterone—a hormone then as rare as estrogen. After months of lonely wanderings and feverish activity in a makeshift lab set up in a garden shed, he finally produced a jarful of progesterone, worth about $160,000 at the time. This was more progesterone than anyone in the world had ever seen in a single batch.

In 1943, the former professor, then forty years old, rough and shabby looking from his sojourn in the wilderness, took his jar down to Mexico City and casually set it down on the desk of the president of a small chemical company founded shortly before by two Hungarian refugees. The Hungarians immediately realized that Marker had broken the market in progesterone, and, after a few days of wild bargaining, Marker and the Hungarians came to an agreement that resulted in a new firm—Snytex Sociedad Anonima—which revolutionalized the entire field of sex hormones. By 1945, the retail price of progestins had fallen by almost half, and physicians everywhere were now able to prescribe these hormones to patients who never before could afford the treatment. This was the great economic turning point in the history of hormone therapy.

To Russell Marker, however, success brought little satisfaction and no rest. He didn't feel at home in gleaming laboratories. He preferred working alone in a little shed in the backyard of the new plant. Soon after, he sold out his interest in the firm and disappeared. Pharmaceutical firms throughout the world are still searching for him, hoping to interest this brilliant mind in their projects. Occasionally there is a rumor that Dr. Marker has been seen in some tiny Mexican village. But his trail has never been found. Nobody knows what became of him, whether he is dead or alive.

But, to this day, Indians throughout the Mexican highlands gather the lily roots that are made into progesterone and progestin by Dr. Marker's process. Mainly because of him, the hormone therapy discussed in this book is now within financial reach of nearly every woman. Though chemical techniques have been considerably refined since Dr. Marker first devised the principles of progesterone production, it is still largely due to him that it has been possible to reduce the total cost of oral fertility control to $2.25 per month per woman.

While speaking of the economics of "the pill," I cannot help drawing a parallel—or rather a contrast—between the billions of public money now spent on a projected moon journey and the financing of biological research, whose benefits are palpable to anyone who goes to see a doctor. Dr. Marker's initial working capital in Mexico was a handful of pesos from his personal savings. The development of the fertility control pill—perhaps the most significant discovery of our era—began with a piddling private grant of $2,100 from the Planned Parenthood Foundation—barely enough to pay for the rabbits needed in the first few months of experiments. When one compares the research budgets allocated to exploring celestial bodies with the funds available for increasing our knowledge of the human body, one can't help being struck by the disproportion.

Many doctors and researchers involved with the new methods of fertility control may wish that their discoveries were accepted simply as a useful medical technique, without any fuss raised on non-medical grounds. The decision on whether or not to employ a certain medical technique usually is a matter between the patient and his or her doctor, and no third party interferes in the medical relationship. In the area of fertility control—which should be one of the most private of all medical areas—a third party always seems to be looking through the keyhole: public opinion. As long as the pressure of public opinion is applied in this area, it seems essential that this opinion should be properly informed. A vast educational effort is therefore needed. I do not imply that this education should necessarily favor fertility control. I merely believe that all pertinent knowledge should be freely brought to light so that each couple can make the decision according to their own conscience and in full awareness of the facts.

It should be emphasized, for instance, that the so-called birth control pills are not actually contraceptives. Nothing blocks the male sperm, no artificial device hinders its free passage, and no foreign objects are inserted into the female genitals. The term contraceptive is somewhat of a misnomer, and religious scruples against the use of contraceptive devices therefore need not necessarily apply against "the pill."

At this writing, no official pronouncement has been made on this subject by ecclesiastic authorities of the Catholic Church. It should be kept in mind that the pill simply creates a condition of non-ovulation. It is therefore not illogical to consider the use of anti-ovulent pills as an extension of the "rhythm method"— intercourse during non-ovulation periods.

Whenever I mention fertility control pills in lectures, discussion groups, and forums, somebody in the audience nearly always brings up questions of ethics and morality. I usually point out that I am no better qualified to make moral judgments than the next man, and I certainly do not believe that I have any right to impose my views on anyone else. I am a member of the Catholic Church, but I do not dismiss as necessarily invalid the sincere convictions of other thoughtful men. When I speak of birth control, therefore, I claim no authority other than that of a physician and a responsible member of human society.

As a physician, however, I am constantly aware of the lasting misery that results from an unwanted birth. I think not only of young girls who "have to marry" the wrong boy simply because of a biological accident, or who—unwilling to make such a compromise—bear their child in solitary despair. I think of the countless happy mothers who suddenly find the lives of their whole family thrown into turmoil by the unexpected arrival of another child. Perhaps the most succinct statement concerning unexpected children came from a housewife in her late thirties: "I have five children," she said. "The first three I wanted. They are a joy. The last two I didn't want. They are a tragedy." The chief victim of such a tragedy, I believe, is often the child himself.

It has been charged that the sheer simplicity of using contraceptive pills may spur promiscuity. From the viewpoint of practical medicine, one should rather keep in mind the meaning of birth control for responsible married women. Their object is not promiscuity. Rather it is to protect the children they already have from the added burden of additional children the family cannot afford. What is foremost in their minds is their children's chance for a good education, good housing, and a decent standard of living—hardly reprehensible motives.

No one interested in family planning can overlook the significance of new advances in this field in terms of worldwide demography. Experts have testified before the U.S. Congress that devastating war is unavoidable unless the population pressure is checked in some of the world's more thickly settled countries. According to recent surveys, the benefits of nearly $70,000,000,000 spent by the United States in foreign aid are largely mullified by the population explosion. In the Western hemisphere, particularly, economic progress cannot keep up with the birth rate, and the poor countries—despite aid from the U.S.—are constantly growing poorer and more desperate.

When such statistics are translated into human terms one may visualize Honduran mothers too poor to buy blankets, carrying their newborn babies wrapped in old newspapers. In Nicaragua, for instance, nearly two-thirds of all children never even receive elementary schooling—simply for lack of funds. They thus continue the cycle of uncontrolled fertility, poverty, illiteracy, hunger, disease, and ultimate disaster.

Ask any gynecologist or obstetrician what he considers the worst part of his job, and he will offer just one answer: those dreadful occasions when a doctor must tell a husband of the death of his wife.

The mortality rate in pregnancy and childbirth, fortunately, has been drastically reduced by medical progress in this century. But the death rate from illegal abortions, especially those performed by irresponsible bunglers, is appallingly high. Thousands of women—no one knows how many—die every year as the result of improperly performed abortions. I particularly remember one woman of about forty, who despite her desperate condition on arrival at the hospital was still able to talk. Her husband had brought her in after she complained to him of high fever and abdominal pain. She told me that she had had an illegal abortion because she already had two grown children and did not want another baby at her age. Pathological examination showed that she had not actually been pregnant. Apparently she had been deceived by some menstrual irregularity common in pre-menopausal women. It also showed that the inept abortionist had clumsily pushed his curette through the uterine wall and had pulled an intestinal loop into the uterine cavity without bothering to repair the damage. The result was a general peritonitis which killed the woman after two weeks of frightful suffering.

She had never told her husband the cause of her illness, and I wish I could have spared him the details. But the cause of death had to be stated on the records. I could not conceal it from the distraught husband. At least I did not have to tell him the bitter irony of the fact that the woman had never been pregnant at all.

Tragedies such as these happen every day. Certainly, every physician, every lawmaker, every clergyman, and, most importantly, every woman owes this subject a great deal of serious thought.

In my opinion, no moral or religious problem of any sort is involved when a physician prescribes birth control pills as a treatment for menopausal symptoms, irregular menstruation, or sexual underdevelopment. It then becomes a purely medical matter.

Taken simply as a therapeutic prescription, estrogenic birth control pills bestow triple benefits: 1) they relieve estrogen deficiency and the associated menopausal symptoms; 2) they assure regularity of menstruation; 3) they provide probable protection against breast and genital cancers thanks to keeping the women estrogen-rich.

Indeed, a woman taking birth control pills for menopause prevention may well think of them in that light rather than as contraceptives. Eventually, however, her doctor may want to switch to the type of menopause therapy which alternates estrogen and a progestin at different times of her cycle to maintain a more natural sequence of events.

NOTE: Although the pills proved effective in 93 per cent of cases, it should be noted that the number of patients involved was small. There is still much room for additional study in this field.

10

A Personal Aside

I BELIEVE THAT a doctor's need to know something about his patient is matched by the patient's need to know something about his doctor. The ideal doctor-patient relationship is a personal one, and, like all personal relationships, mutual to some degree. When interviewing a patient about her personal history I have often sensed the patient's wish to ask me the same kind of questions. I have never resented this unspoken, though evident, curiosity. After all, it is only natural for a woman who entrusts herself to my care and judgment to want to know what manner of man I am.

Readers of this book may well feel a similar curiosity about the man speaking to them through these pages; and, while it is rarely possible for a physician to reveal something of himself to his patients, an author may permit himself a few personal remarks. The autobiographic discursions in this chapter are not for the sake of self-aggrandizement, but rather to give my readers some feeling of personal contact with the doctor whom they have consulted through the pages of this book.

My boyhood during the final years of the last century was spent in Ramsbottom, a small town in Lancashire, England, where my father was chief chemist in a small chemical plant. He had achieved this modest eminence entirely by his own efforts, having been born the son of a poor stonecutter. At the age of six, my father was sent to work the looms in one of those grim mills that dotted the sooty towns of Victorian England and which spun the wealth of the rising middle class. By dint of tireless self-education, haunting lectures and libraries, he acquired a professional knowledge of chemistry and engineering, and he also taught himself German, French, Italian, and Russian. So equipped, and fired by the kind of tireless intellectual curiosity that is the natural endowment of the most fortunate among men, he eventually devised a number of patents that enabled him to escape the drudgery of the mills and in later years set up his own business.

In these few lines devoted to the memory of my father, I should serve him ill to stress merely his technical and business acumen. For, in an era marked by the astounding narrow-mindedness of men who believed that the Glory of the Empire was the peak of Christian civilization, my father stubbornly maintained the kind of refreshing independence of mind that—to his contemporaries—marked him as a "radical."

My lifelong involvement with women—or rather the

idea of feminity—dates back to those boyhood days. I still recall a chubby, plain-faced little girl named Madge Morris who came up to me in the school yard when I was about seven or eight years old. "Will you be my sweetheart?" she asked.

I didn't quite know what the word meant, but she had asked in so kind a voice that I immediately said yes. Then she kissed me.

Perhaps the fondness of this recollection misleads me, but I believe that my lifelong penchant for the more magic attributes of love stems from that moment. If, in the routine of clinical gynecology, I have been able to maintain a firm belief in the sanctity and the miracle of love between the sexes, some of the credit belongs to the wonderfully innocent emotional generosity of that little girl.

Other happenings predestined my career. One was the tragic decline of my gentle and almost angelic mother. At the time I could not understand it. What was a boy in his teens to make of a phrase like "change of life"—especially if it was spoken in the tone of voice that in those days was used to mention any number of things then considered unmentionable. How could anything connected with my mother be spoken of in that tone of voice? Yet something terrible was obviously happening. I was appalled at the transformation of that vital, wonderful woman who had been the dynamic focal point of our family into a pain-racked, petulant invalid. I could feel the deep wounds her senseless rages inflicted on my father, myself, and the younger children. It was this frightful experience that later directed my interest as a physician to the problem of menopause.

One event, in particular, impressed on me the horrors of menopause. Near the outskirts of Ramsbottom was a small reservoir circled by a stone wall where I often used to play. One day I noticed several men bending over the wall, shouting excitedly to each other. I ran close, and in their preoccupation with fishing a drowned woman's body out of the water, none of the men noticed me, and none took me away. Thus I was left to witness the terrible moment when one of the grappling hooks ripped an enormous gash in the bloated corpse. The sheer horror of it haunted me for months.

Why had she drowned herself? "Gone mad," the town gossips insisted. "The change of life," they added by way of explanation.

That phrase again! And in bewildered innocence I made a dreadful mental connection between the ripped body of the drowned woman and my own mother.

Slowly this event receded in my mind. By the time my father had moved the family to the United States for business reasons I hardly ever thought of it. But it may well be that the episode at Ramsbottom Reservoir remained alive in my unconscious mind, guiding me toward the choice of my medical specialty and my particular area of research.

The power of subconscious motivation also became

evident as a guiding factor at a crucial point in my later career. One of the key elements in the development of menopause therapy emerged quite obviously from the hidden regions of my mind, thus bearing out current theories as to the nature of the creative imagination. By that time I had become deeply engrossed in estrogen research, but had not yet found a fully successful form of therapy. I had established to my own satisfaction that estrogen relieved menopausal symptoms. But too many women under treatment were troubled by irregular and often severe and persistent bleeding.

I spent my days poring over charts listing dosage and timing variations, hoping to discern some pattern by which the benefits of estrogen might be obtained without untoward side effects. One night as I fell asleep, my mind was still struggling with these problems. In an ensuing dream I saw myself counting up the days in a patient's menstrual cycle and then jotting one word on the calendar: PROGESTIN.

Guided by my subconscious, I had hit upon the principle that made estrogen therapy truly practicable: the alternation of estrogen and one of the newly-discovered progestins to simulate the natural sequence of the hormonal cycle.

The years that followed were devoted to working out the details of timing and dosage that made this dream-inspired therapy ultimately successful.

During this period of intensive research work, my energies were sustained by the deep and profound satisfaction of a happy marriage and a rewarding family life. To balance my absorption in professional matters, I made a point of cultivating other interests, particularly in music and such sports as hiking and golf. One sport in particular I found tremendously thrilling. The idea of flying had always appealed to me, and though I obtained my pilot's license rather late in life, I developed sufficient skill to go in for the kind of aerial acrobatics usually reserved for professional stunt flyers.

My greatest pleasure however, was the acquisition of a magnificent classic Mercedes 540 K cabriolet. My choice of this car goes back to a boyhood experience in Ramsbottom which was overwhelming to me at the time. I am sure that it shaped certain attitudes I carried with me throughout life. On the surface, what happened may seem very trivial. It is simply that one afternoon a glorious motorcar passed through our town. With its supercharger screaming, its radiator pointing forward like the prow of a great ship, its high fenders outlining the wheels in a gesture of graceful caress, this vintage Mercedes embodied a sense of beauty and adventure totally lacking in the impersonally efficient tin boxes that today swamp our highways.

It would be difficult to say exactly what the appearance of that car meant to me as a boy. But it was a vision that might perhaps be compared to the experiencing of a great work of art. To me it was a lifting of the sense toward undreamed-of horizons where the great elements of creative design converge—where form and function, grace and power merge into the feeling of joy.

The car I bought as a grown man was an updated replica of the one that had so enchanted me as a boy.

I often wondered why this motorcar should have given me such a mental lift, such a wonderful sense of emotional buoyancy. After all, I was no longer a child to be charmed by a toy, nor the kind of man who needed expensive possessions to assure himself of his own worth. My best guess is that that car—in some deep region of my mind—was to me a mistress.

Man is by nature polygamous, a fact which most non-European civilizations have always calmly and openly recognized. A great deal of human misery stems from the failure of our culture to do likewise. Wives have no culturally "normal" way of coping emotionally with a husband's philandering. They think of it as infidelity. In truth, an extramarital affair may not, in the literal sense of the term, involve any infidelity at all. For a man may loyally maintain a deep love for his wife and yet feel the need for a kind of thrill that a wife with her aura of comfortable domesticity cannot give. Thus the paradoxical situation arises that a husband may go astray in search of casual encounters *just because* he is happy and comfortable with his wife!

But as long as jealousy remains one of the basic human emotions, how can this civilization provide some suitable outlet for the male impulse toward polygamy? The answer, I believe, is that the source from which a man obtains certain emotional thrills need not necessarily be another woman. If he has a normal, happy sex life with his wife, he can direct his need for self-assertion and conquest toward some absorbing challenge—a field of study, a hobby, a sport— something that arouses his energies, satisfies his sense of beauty, and stimulates his sense of adventure. For me, it was my Mercedes, which satisfied the hidden longing implanted on the boyhood afternoon many years earlier when that great touring car roared into Ramsbottom.

But not even the possession of that car, nor the other comforts and pleasures deriving from outward success, could quite subdue a nagging kind of unrest. I felt thwarted in what I considered the most vital area of my work. An increasing number of cases bore evidence that the methods of treating the menopause and its aftermath were both safe and effective. There was no longer any possible doubt that I had developed a medical procedure of tremendous value to every woman. Yet it was most difficult to interest anyone in these discoveries. With leading medical journals indifferent to my papers, there seemed little hope of reaching other members of my profession, let alone the millions of women who might directly benefit from my work.

I consoled myself for a seemingly endless sequence of frustrations by reflecting on the fate of other medical innovators. In particular my thoughts dwelt on Dr. Ignaz Semmelweiss, the shy, kindly Austrian doctor who in the middle of the last century—long before Pasteur—had recognized the fact of contagion. "Gentlemen," Semmelweiss urged his colleagues, "if you would just wash your hands between examining different patients, I believe you could reduce the spread of infection."

At first the response was simply laughter at such an outrageous notion. Preventing illness by simply washing one's hands—ridiculous. But soon the dumb anger of unthinking incompetence arose against Semmelweiss. "How dare he suggest that doctors can cause infection?" fulminated Vienna's eminent professors. They fired Semmelweiss from his post and ran him out of the city which—thanks partly to him—was soon afterward to become one of the world's great centers of medical learning.

But Semmelweiss never lived to see the vindication of his prophetic ideas. Crushed by the ruin of his career and the personal humiliation heaped upon him, he ended his life in an asylum for the insane.

I thought of Jenner, who conceived the idea of inoculation, of Pasteur and his theory that germs might be disease carriers, and finally of the man whose work was so closely allied to my own, Dr. George N. Papanicolaou, the originator of the Pap Test. All these men had been rebuffed by the medical authorities of their time, and their private disappointments were made even more bitter by the despairing thought that countless lives might have been saved but for the mental sloth and obstinacy that for so long opposed the adoption of their methods.

In studying the lives of these physicians, I had no wish—not even subconsciously—to compare myself to these great men. My object was to understand the historic process by which the knowledge of new medical discoveries is spread in the profession, and to defend myself psychologically against the disappointments and delays which I was experiencing.

As a physician, I realized that the traditional skepticism with which the medical profession receives new discoveries is, in fact, a valuable protection for the public. Certainly it would be foolhardy for physicians to welcome novelty for its own sake. Scientific method is always slow and ponderous, but its insistence upon rigorous proof is our best assurance of ultimate truth. The personal frustrations visited upon the innovator, I told myself, do not really count in the long run.

As I devoted more time to research and writing and less to my private practice, my income shrank from a very comfortable sum that had allowed me many pleasures and luxuries to one that required a good deal of tight budgeting. And I cannot deny that on the day I sold my beautiful Mercedes in order to continue my work, I felt that I had indeed joined the company of the martyrs of science.

With the loyal help of a small circle of co-workers and "converts," I was eventually able to present the modern views on menopause to larger medical groups, and general acceptance of hormone therapy now

seems imminent at last. As I retire from active practice, I shall continue to devote myself to research
under the auspices of organizations established to
further the cause of menopause treatment, and I am
now happy in the knowledge that my work has led to
some ultimate good.

As long as I am permitted to address my readers on
this very personal level, I should like to touch very
briefly on a matter of philosophy that I believe essential to medical and all other research.

I have never understood why some people feel that
to know nature is to offend God. Among the reactions I
encounter I still come across those persons who would
tear the telescope from Galileo's eyes or wrest the dis-
secting knife from the hand of Vesalius. Such persons
may be no less sincere in their search for enlightenment, but they seek for some miracle outside of nature; they forget that nature itself is the greatest miracle. In learning to know nature, we learn to know
something of God. And scientific research, if under-
taken in this spirit, is a form of worship.

11

A Salute to Tomorrow's Woman

WE STAND AT a threshold. Like Moses glimpsing the Promised Land, we can today see the outlines of a world in which—unless nuclear war destroys our civilization—life's possibilities are multiplied a thousandfold. Only within this generation have the benefits of technology begun to enrich the lives of great numbers of people. The possibilities of modern travel are opening the world to the average citizen, at least in America and Europe. New means of communication provide us with undreamed-of plentitudes of information and of art, and it is surely only a matter of time until such media as radio and worldwide television will, in addition to mere entertainment, offer increasingly worthwhile options to the mind.

The basic process of useful work is being transformed before our eyes by the growth of automation, promising new dimensions of creative leisure if the economic aspects of this change can be intelligently planned.

Among the great possibilities of the future, the elimination of menopause takes on added significance. Seen in historic perspective, the technique of menopause prevention reaches far beyond the scope of any single life. It means that, for the first time in history, women may share the promise of tomorrow as biological equals of men. Specifically, they can remain able and active in mind and body for their entire lives. Thanks to hormone therapy, they may look forward to prolonged well-being and extended youth.

The Wilson Research Foundation, of which I am President, will provide additional information on the subject of menopause prevention to any woman seeking it as well as professional information to any doctor who inquires. It is located at 777 Third Avenue in New York City.

Recognizing menopause as a curable deficiency disease rather than as an inexorable fate, as we have pointed out, carries widespread implications—physical, mental, and cultural. To summarize them briefly, allow me to point once more to some of the main arguments set forth in this book:

1. Menopause is unnecessary. It can be prevented entirely. Younger women need never experience it. And older women can in most cases be assured almost complete recovery from their symptoms.

2. Preventive treatment should begin, preferably during the middle thirties, before the onset of menopause. This will forestall any of the usual physical changes associated with menopause.

3. The myth that estrogen is a causative factor in cancer has been proven to be entirely false. On the contrary, indications are that estrogen acts as a cancer preventive. Certainly the continuance of regular menstruation throughout life has a healthful cleansing effect on uterine tissues and seemingly reduces the incidence of uterine cancer.

4. Menopausal symptoms, such as weakening of bones and muscles, dowager's hump, gastro-intestinal disorders, heart trouble, hardening of the arteries, atrophy of the breasts and sexual organs, disturbed vision, wrinkling of the skin, pains in the joints, etc., can be avoided by pre-menopausal therapy and often cured by post-menopausal therapy.

5. The mental depression typical of so many menopausal women can be avoided by early treatment and often greatly alleviated even in obstinate cases. Difficult family situations can often be wholly remedied by estrogen therapy for the woman involved.

6. Sexual competence and enjoyment can now be assured to women long past middle age. Many difficult marital situations can thus be happily resolved.

7. Youthful appearance and vigorous energy can be

retained through estrogen therapy for decades beyond the customary age of menopausal decline.

8. And, bear in mind, the use of estrogen-progestin therapy will not prolong fertility by a single day.

With these enormous benefits at her disposal, I hope that the woman of the future will value her essential femininity more highly than ever, and that it will serve as a humanizing influence on future generations. Since hormone therapy will enable women to maintain their full femininity throughout life, the effect of their femininity will proportionately increase.

This thought opens vistas of a "sexual revolution" in a far broader sense than a mere change in social mores. The greater influence of the feminine element in human society may herald a new stage in the evolution of human sensibilities. It may yet turn mankind toward more peaceful, more beautiful, and more rewarding ways of life.

Assured of her lasting femininity, and no longer defensive about her womanliness, tomorrow's woman may instill new values and attitudes in her children, and these attitudes may eventually permeate the entire structure of our civilization. Tomorrow's woman, far more so than any of her forebears, may realize the ultimate mission of her sex: to broaden the role of love as an operative agent in human affairs.

If women are destined to accomplish this, it must be through proud recognition of their distinctly feminine qualities. My hope is that the medical procedures outlined in this book will provide a physical and mental aid toward the attainment and lifelong preservation of that precious femininity. To those women of the future, I dedicate my work and offer my salute.

Medical Appendix

A Complete List of Dr. Wilson's Degrees, Affiliations, and Associations

Consultant in Obstetrics and Gynecology, Methodist Hospital, Brooklyn, N.Y.

Consultant in Obstetrics and Gynecology, St. Mary's Hospital, Brooklyn, N.Y.

Consultant in Obstetrics and Gynecology, Putnam Community Hospital, Carmel, N.Y.

Diplomate of the American Board of Obstetrics and Gynecology

Diplomate of the International College of Surgeons

Fellow of the American College of Surgeons

Fellow of the International College of Surgeons

Founder-Fellow of the American College of Obstetricians and Gynecologists

Fellow of the American Geriatrics Society

Fellow of the New York Academy of Medicine
Fellow of the New York Gynecological Society
Life-Fellow of the Brooklyn Gynecological Society
Fellow of the American Medical Association and the
    Medical Society of the State of New York
Member of the American Fertility Society
Member of the American Society of Cytology
Member of the International Fertility Association
Member of the Pan-American Medical Association
Member of the Gerontological Society
Member of the Society for the Advancement of Science
Member of the American Medical Writers Association
President, The Wilson Research Foundation, New
    York, N.Y.

Bibliography

PHYSICIANS ARE referred to the following sources on menopausal therapy and related aspects.

1. Wilson, R.A., and Wilson, T.A.: "The Fate of the Nontreated Postmenopausal Woman: A Plea for the Maintenance of Adequate Estrogen from Puberty to the Grave," *J. Am. Geriatrics Soc.* 11:347-362 (Apr.) 1963.
2. Wilson, R.A., Brevetti, R.E., and Wilson, T.A.: "Specific Procedures for the Elimination of the Menopause," *Western J. Surg., Obst. & Gynec.* 71:110-121 (May-June) 1963.
3. Wilson, R.A.: "The Obsolete Menopause," Editorial, *Connecticut Medicine* 27:735 (Dec.) 1963.
4. Wilson, R.A.: "The Menopause is Obsolete," Editorial, *Northwest Medicine*, p. 943 (Dec.) 1963.
5. Wilson, R.A.: "Menopause—Method of Robert A. Wilson, M.D.," *Current Therapy*, 1965, p. 661.
6. Wilson, R.A., Marino, E.R., Wilson, T.A., and Wilson, G.I.: "The Treatment of the Perimenopause," *Excerpta Medica Foundation*, pp. 32-36, 1965: Proceedings of the Symposium on Female Reproductive Physiology, Sept. 12, 1964, Birmingham, Alabama.
7. Wilson, R.A.: "Estrogen Administration Beyond the Menopause Regardless of the Presence or Absence of the Uterus," *Ob-Gyn Collected Letters*, Series IV, p. 157 (Oct. 15) 1963.
8. Wilson, R.A.: "Use of Oral Contraceptive after Age of Forty," *Ob-Gyn Collected Letters*, Series V, p. 111 (July) 1964.
9. Wilson, R.A., Marino, E.R., and Wilson, T.A.: "Norethynodrel-Mestranol for Prevention and Treatment of the Perimenopause," in press.

Bibliography

10. Wilson, R.A.: "The Roles of Estrogen and Progesterone in Breast and Genital Cancer," *J.A.M.A.* 182:327-331 (Oct. 27) 1962.
11. Wilson, R.A.: "Breast and Genital Cancer," *Yearbook of Cancer* 1963-1964 Series, pp. 77-78.
12. Wilson, R.A.: "Adequate Estrogen from Puberty to the Grave," *Yearbook of Cancer* 1963-1964 Series, pp. 213-214.
13. Wilson, R.A.: "The Estrogen Cancer Myth," *Clinical Medicine,* 71:1343-1352 (Aug.) 1964.

14. Hobbs, J.E.: "The Climacterium," *Current Med. Digest* 26:57-66 (May) 1959.
15. Greenblatt, R.B.: "Metabolic and Psychosomatic Disorders in Menopausal Women," *Geriatrics* 10:165-169 (Apr.) 1955.
16. Masters, W.H.: "Sex Steroid Influence on the Aging Process," *Am. J. Obst. & Gynec.* 74:733-746 (Oct.) 1957.
17. Shorr, E.: "The Menopause," *Bulletin.* New York Acad. Med. 16:453-474 (July) 1940.
18. Wiesbader, H., and Kurzrok, R.: "The Menopause: A Consideration of the Symptoms, Etiology, and Treatment by Means of Estrogens," *Endocrinology* 23:32-38 (July) 1938.
19. Malleson, J.: a) "An Endocrine Factor in Certain Affective Disorders," *Lancet* 2:158-164 (July 25) 1953; b) "Climacteric Stress: Its Empirical Management," *Brit. M.J.* 2:1422-1425 (Dec. 15) 1956.
20. Hamblen, E.C.: "Geriatric Gynecology," in Stieglitz, E.J.: *Geriatric Medicine,* ed. 2. Phila., W.B. Saunders Company, 1949, Chap. 41, pp. 657-673.
21. Masters, W.H.: "The Female Reproductive System," in Lansing, A.I.: *Cowdrey's Problems of Aging: Biological and Medical Aspects,* ed. 3. Baltimore, The Williams & Wilkins Company, 1952, pp. 651-685.
22. Kirk, J.E.: "Steroid Hormones and Aging: A Review," *J. Gerontol.* 6:253-262 (July) 1951.
23. Heller, A.L., and Shipley, R.A.: "Endocrine Studies in Aging" (Read before the Second Internat. Gerontol. Congress, St. Louis, Sept. 9-14, 1951), *Abstr. J. Gerontol.* (suppl. 3) 6:101 (July) 1951.
24. Cronqvist, M., and Kullander, S.: "Norethynodrel Effect after

Menopause," *Acta Obst. et Gynec. Scandinav.*, 40:43-58 (Fasc. 1), 1961.

25. Herschberg, A.D.: "The Receptivity to Estrogens after the Climacteric," *Rev. franc. Gerontol.*, 5:281, 1959; through Excerpta Med. Sec. 20 (*Gerontol. & Geriatrics*) 4:89, (Feb.) 1961.

26. Solez, C.: "Aging and Adrenal Cortical Hormones," *Geriatrics* 7:290-294 (Sept., Oct.) 1952.

27. Frommer, D.J.: "Changing Age of Menopause," *Brit. Med. J.* 2:349-351 (Aug. 8) 1964.

28. Kinch, R.A.H., et al.: "Primary Ovarian Failure," *Am. J. Obst. & Gynec.* 91:630-644 (Mar. 1) 1965.

29. Keetel, W.C., and Bradbury, J.T.: "Premature Ovarian Failure, Permanent and Temporary," *Am. J. Obst. & Gynec.* 89:83-96 (May) 1964.

30. Goldberg, M.B.: "Medical Management of the Menopause," *Mod. Med. Monographs,* Grune & Stratton, New York, 1959, p. 60.

31. Pratt, J.P.: "Gynecologic Problems of Aging," *Postgrad. Med.* 37:214-215 (Feb.) 1965.

32. McEwen, D.C.: "Ovarian Failure and the Menopause," *The Canadian Med. Assoc. J.* 92:962-969 (May 1) 1965.

33. Bakke, J.L.: "A Double-Blind Study of a Progestin-Estrogen Combination in the Management of the Menopause," *Pac. Med. & Surg.* 73:200-205 (May-June) 1965.

34. Drill, V.A.: "Endocrine Properties and Long-term Safety of Oral Contraceptives," *Metabolism* 14:305 (Mar.) 1965.

35. Lin, TaJung, and Lin, Su-Chin: "The Vaginal Cytogram, A Guide to Substitution Therapy for States of Ovarian Deficiency," *J.A.M.A.* 185:844-849, 1963.

36. Toth, F., and Gimes, R.: "Sections at Autopsy Compared with Smears Made in Life," *Zeitschrift für Geburtshilfe und Gynakologie* 160; 3:251, 1965.

37. Moyer, D.L., Tyler, E.T., Olsen, H.J., and Zeldis, L.J.: "Vaginal Cytohormonal Effects in Long-term Cyclic Administration of Synthetic Progestins," *Fertil. & Steril.* 15:170-172 (Mar. Apr.) 1964.

38. Pincus, G., and Garcia, C.-R.: "Studies on Vaginal, Cervical and Uterine Histology," *Metabolism* 14:436 (Mar.) 1965.

39. Liu, W.: "Correlation Between Vaginal Cytology and Endo-

Bibliography

metrial Histology," *Amer. J. Obst. & Gynec.* 80:321-324 (Aug.) 1960.

40. Nesbitt, R.E.L., Jr. et al.: "The Prognostic Value of Vaginal Cytology in Pregnancy," *Obst. & Gynec.* 17:2-8 (Jan.) 1961.

41. Rakoff, A.E.: "Hormonal Cytology in Gynecology," in *Clinical Obstetrics and Gynecology*, Edited by K.P. Russell and A.E. Rakoff, Hoeber-Harper, New York, December 1961, Vol. IV, pp. 1045-1059.

42. Smith, O.W., Smith, G.V., and Gavian, N.G.: "Urinary Estrogens in Women," *Amer. J. Obst. & Gynec.* 78:1028-1047 (Nov.) 1959.

43. Pedersen-Bjergaard, K., and Tonnessen, M.: Oestrogenic Androgenic and Gonadotrophic Substances in the Urine of Normal Women, *Acta Endocrinol.* 1:38-60, 1948.

44. Paulsen, C.A., and Others: "Function of the Postmenopausal Ovary. Comparison of Urinary Estrogen and Gonadotropin Excretion and Response to Administration of FSH in Postmenopausal and Ovariectomized Women," *J. Am. Geriatrics Soc.* 6:803-813 (Nov.) 1958.

45. Stoll, P.: "Androgenic Effect on Vaginal Epithelial Cells: The Effect of Physiological Sex Hormones on the Vaginal Epithelium of Patients with Inactive Ovaries," *Acta Cytolog.* 1:77, 1957.

46. De Alvarez, R.R., and Smith, E.K.: "Physiological Basis for Hormone Therapy in the Female," *J.A.M.A.* 168:489-495 (Oct. 4) 1958.

47. Russ, E.M., Eder, H.A., and Barr, D.P.: "Influence of Gonadal Hormones on Protein-Lipid Relationships in Human Plasma," *Am. J. Med.* 19:4-24 (July) 1955.

48. Jeffcoate, T.N.A.: "Oestrogenic Hormone Therapy," *Brit. Med. J.* 2:671-676 (Sept. 30) 1939.

49. Griffith, G.C.: "Oöphorectomy and Cardiovascular Tissues," *Obst. & Gynec.* 7:479-482 (May) 1956.

50. Taylor, R.D., Corcoran, A.C., and Page, I.H.: "Menopausal Hypertension: A Critical Study," *Am. J. M. Sc.* 213:475-476 (Apr.) 1947.

51. Wuest, J.H., Jr., Dry, T.J., and Edwards, J.E.: "The Degree of Coronary Atherosclerosis in Bilaterally Oöphorectomized Women," *Circulation* 7:801-809 (June) 1953.

52. Marmorston, J., Magidson, O., Lewis, J.J., Mehl, J., Moore, F.J., and Bernstein, J.: "Effect of Small Doses of Estrogen on Serum

Lipids in Female Patients with Myocardial Infarction," *New England J. Med.* 258:583-586 (Mar. 20) 1958.

53. Davis, M.E., Jones, R.J., and Jarolim, C.: "Long-term Estrogen Substitution and Atherosclerosis," *Am. J. Obst. & Gynec.* 82: 1003-1018 (Nov.) 1961.

54. Robinson, R.W., Cohen, W.D., and Higano, N.: "Clinical and Serum Lipid Effects of a Combination of Norethynodrel plus Ethynylestradiol 3-methyl Ether in Postmenopausal Women," *The Am. J. Med. Sc.* 244:736-743 (Dec.) 1962.

55. Reifenstein, E.C., Jr.: "Osteoporosis," in Harrison, T.R.: *Principles of Internal Medicine*, ed. 3. New York, The Blakiston Division, McGraw-Hill Book Company, Inc., 1958, pp. 664-671.

56. Gessler, C.J., Halsted, J.A., and Stetson, R.P.: "Effect of Estrogenic Substance on Blood Sugar of Female Diabetics After the Menopause," *J. Clin. Invest.* 18:715-722 (Nov.) 1939.

57. Cohen, A., Dubbs, A.W., and Myers, A.: "Treatment of Atrophic Arthritis with Estrogenic Substances," *New England J. Med.* 222:140-142 (Jan. 25) 1940.

58. Drant, P.H.: "Endocrine Factors in Dermatology," *Pennsylvania M. J.* 52:966-974 (June) 1949.

59. Dynes, J.B.: "Estrogenic Therapy of Involutional Melancholia," *Arch. Neurol. & Psychiat.* 42:248-259 (Aug.) 1939.

60. Strauss, J.S., and Poch, P.E.: "Effect of Cyclic Progestin-Estrogen Therapy on Sebum and Acne in Women," *J.A.M.A.* 190: 815-819 (Nov.) 1964.

61. Swanson, D.W., et al.: "Norethynodrel Used in Psychotic Women," *Am. J. Psych.* 120:1101-1103, 1964.

62. Strauss, J.S., and Kligman, A.M.: "Androgenic Effects of Progestational Compound, 17 a-ethynyl-19-noretestosterone (Norlutin) on Human Sebaceous Gland," *J. Clin. Endocr.* 21:215-219 (Feb.) 1961.

63. Sherman, A.L., and Woolf, R.B.: "An Endocrine Basis for Endometrial Carcinoma," *Am. J. Obst. & Gynec.* 77:233-242 (Feb.) 1959.

64. Mustacchi, P., and Gordan, G.S.: "Frequency of Cancer in Estrogen-Treated Osteoporotic Women" (in Segaloff, A.: *Breast Cancer*), The Second Biennial Louisiana Cancer Conference, New Orleans, Jan. 22-23, 1958, The C.V. Mosby Company, St. Louis, 1958, pp. 163-169.

65. Kelley, R.M., and Baker, W.H.: "Progesterone for Endometrial

Bibliography

Carcinoma," *New England J. Med.* 264:216-222 (Apr.) 1961.

66. Huggins, C., Grand, L.C., and Brillantes, F.P.: "Mammary Cancer Induced by Single Feedings of Polynuclear Hydrocarbons," *Nature* (London) 189:204-207 (Jan.) 1961.

67. Bimes, C., Planel, H., and David, J.F.: "Use of Estradiol, Testosterone, Inhibits Malignant Cell Growth," *Med. Tribune,* p. 2 (June 5) 1961.

68. Kistner, R.W.: "Histological Effects of Progestins on Hyperplasia and Carcinoma in situ of the Endometrium," *Cancer,* 12:1106-1122 (Nov.-Dec.) 1959.

69. Alvizouri, M.: "Effect of Progesterone on Experimental Endometrial Hyperplasias," *Am. J. Obst. & Gynec.* 82:1224-1227 (Dec.) 1961.

70. Wallach, S., and Henneman, P.H.: "Prolonged Estrogen Therapy in Postmenopausal Women," *J.A.M.A.* 171:1637-1642 (Nov. 21) 1959.

71. Kistner, R.W.: "Uses of Progestins," *Postgrad. Med.* 35:225-232, 1964.

72. Wentz, W.B.: "Effect of a Progestational Agent on Endometrial Hyperplasia and Endometrial Cancer," *Obst. & Gynec.* 24:370-375, 1964.

73. Stoll, B.A.: "A New Progestational Steroid in the Therapy of Endometrial Carcinoma—A Preliminary Report," *Cancer* Chemother. Rep. No. 14:83-84 (Oct.) 1961.

74. Steiner, G.J., Kistner, R.W., and Craig, J.M.: "Histological Effects of Progestins on Hyperplasia and Carcinoma in situ of the Endometrium—Further Observations," *Metabolism* 14:356-386 (Mar.) 1965.

75. Kennedy, B.J.: "A Progestogin for Treatment of Advanced Endometrial Cancer," *J.A.M.A.* 184:758-761, 1964.

76. Suminori, H.: "Estrogen Influence on Radiosensitivity of Cervical Cancer Patients," *Hyushu J. Med. Sc.* 14:355-368, 1964.

77. Kistner, R.W.: "Treatment of Carcinoma in situ of the Endometrium," *Clin. Obst. & Gyn.* 5:1166-1180 (Dec.) 1962.

78. Kelley, R.M., and Baker, W.H.: "Progestational Agents in the Treatment of Carcinoma of the Endometrium," *New England J. Med.* 264:216, 1961.

A professional advisory service as well as popularly written educational pamphlets for patients are offered without charge by The Wilson Research Foundation, 777 Third Avenue, New York, N.Y. 10017.

Index